Fundamentals of
Biomedical
Research

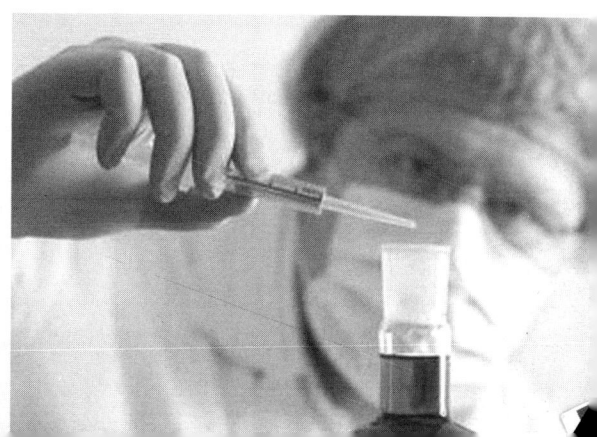

Salient Features of this Edition

- Compressive review of research methods
- Introduction to epidemiological research
- Study designs
- Simple language and lucid style
- Thesis writing
- Paper publication
- Peer review
- Evaluating research papers
- Clinical trials
- Clinical research overview
- Statistical methods
- Glossary for better understanding

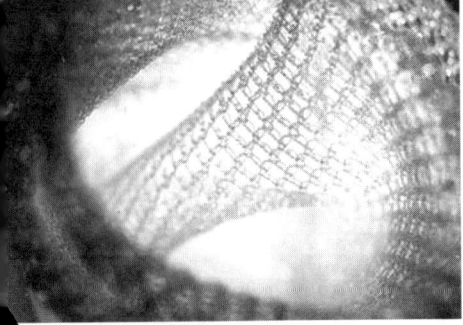

Fundamentals of
Biomedical
Research

Vikas Dhikav

MBBS, MD (3 years, AIIMS), PhD (Neurology, PGIMER, Delhi), PhD (h/c),
Dip Clinical Research, Fellowship CI Neuropsychopharm and
Cognitive Neurology, Honorary Professor, ISM-IUK, Bishkek,
Kyrgyzstan (Erstwhile USSR) & Guangzhou, China

Senior Research Officer
Department of Neurology
Dr RML Hospital and PGIMER
(GGS-IP University)
New Delhi, India

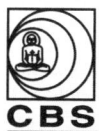

CBS

CBS Publishers & Distributors Pvt Ltd

New Delhi • Bengaluru • Chennai • Kochi • Kolkata • Mumbai
Hyderabad • Jharkhand • Nagpur • Patna • Pune • Uttarakhand

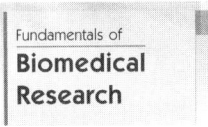

Fundamentals of
Biomedical Research

ISBN: 978-93-87085-86-2

Copyright © Author and Publisher

First Edition: 2018

Published by Satish Kumar Jain and produced by Varun Jain for

CBS Publishers & Distributors Pvt Ltd
4819/XI Prahlad Street, 24 Ansari Road, Daryaganj, New Delhi 110 002, India.
Ph: 23289259, 23266861, 23266867 Website: www.cbspd.com
Fax: 011-23243014   e-mail: delhi@cbspd.com; cbspubs@airtelmail.in.
Corporate Office: 204 FIE, Industrial Area, Patparganj, Delhi 110 092

Ph: 4934 4934   Fax: 4934 4935   e-mail: publishing@cbspd.com; publicity@cbspd.com

Branches

- **Bengaluru:** Seema House 2975, 17th Cross, K.R. Road,
  Banasankari 2nd Stage, Bengaluru 560 070, Karnataka
  Ph: +91-80-26771678/79   Fax: +91-80-26771680   e-mail: bangalore@cbspd.com
- **Chennai:** 7, Subbaraya Street, Shenoy Nagar, Chennai 600 030, Tamil Nadu
  Ph: +91-44-26680620, 26681266   Fax: +91-44-42032115   e-mail: chennai@cbspd.com
- **Kochi:** Ashana House, No. 39/1904, AM Thomas Road, Valanjambalam,
  Ernakulam 682 016, Kochi, Kerala
  Ph: +91-484-4059061-65   Fax: +91-484-4059065   e-mail: kochi@cbspd.com
- **Kolkata:** 6/B, Ground Floor, Rameswar Shaw Road, Kolkata-700 014, West Bengal
  Ph: +91-33-22891126, 22891127, 22891128   e-mail: kolkata@cbspd.com
- **Mumbai:** 83-C, Dr E Moses Road, Worli, Mumbai-400018, Maharashtra
  Ph: +91-22-24902340/41   Fax: +91-22-24902342   e-mail: mumbai@cbspd.com

Representatives

• **Hyderabad**	0-9885175004	• **Jharkhand**	0-9811541605	• **Nagpur**	0-9021734563
• **Patna**	0-9334159340	• **Pune**	0-9623451994	• **Uttarakhand**	0-9716462459

Printed At : Goyal Offset Printers

to

my beloved wife
Meenakshi and Angel Daughters
Priyanshi and Princi

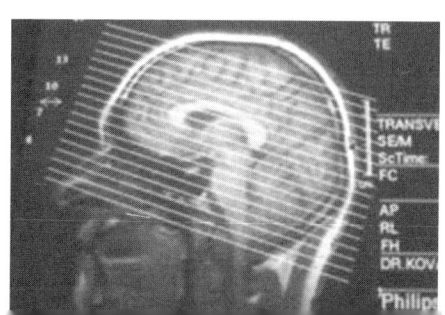

Preface

Majority of medical students, doctors, dentists, scientists, biomedical students and those in biomedical research at advanced levels (e.g. PhDs) find research methodology a difficult topic.

This science can become challenging even to professionals in full-time basic or clinical research at times. I felt the need to have a simple and clearly outlined book so that everyone who is involved in biomedical research, be at graduate or doctoral level, so that one gets a fair understanding of the topic.

The attempt has been made to keep long and complicated mathematical formulae at bay so that the already rampant fear of research methods is kept away. Overall, I have tried to make this dreaded subject an easy going one. The book provides an introduction to the concept of research methods, basic biostatistical methods, biostatistical softwares, publication and research process and the steps needed in research development for students and professionals alike.

Vikas Dhikav

vikasdhikav@hotmail.com

Contents

Introduction to Research

Learning objectives

Understanding "the scientific methods" is needed for understanding the research methodology. The chapter details the outlines about the role of a hypothesis in a research study. Also, detailed are the strategies underlying hypothesis formulation. The chapter ends with the methods/strategies to test statement of a hypothesis.

WHAT IS RESEARCH?

Research is generally defined as, "knowledge acquisition or experience gained via reasoning, intuition but most importantly through the use of appropriate scientific or research methods".

Another way of defining research is "An organized and systematic way to find answers to questions". Importantly, research is a creative process, medical research being no exception. Talking practically, *research* is the application of the scientific method to solve scientific queries. In other words, *it is a systematic process of collecting and logically analyzing information or data.*

As per an online dictionary definition, research is "diligent and systematic inquiry or investigation into a subject in order to discover or revise already known facts, theories, applications, etc.".

Generally speaking it's about something that we want to know about our discipline, or about a specific area within our discipline, e.g. why does joint pain occur in chikungunya fever or why do platelet counts drop in dengue fever, etc.

It is important to note that research is not a topic, fragment, phrase, or sentence. So it begins with a question (research question) and it ends with a question mark (Fig. 1.1)!

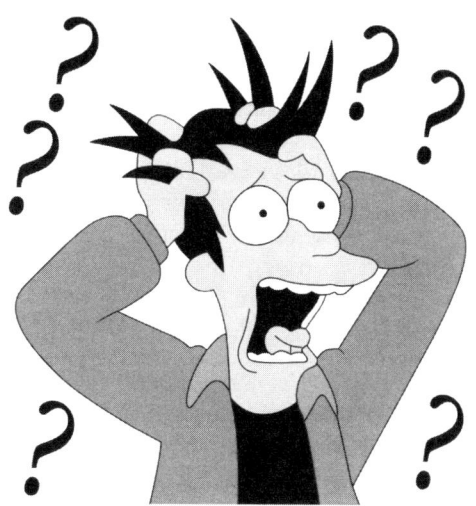

Fig. 1.1: Research starts with a question and ends with questions

WHY DO RESEARCH?

Knowledge obtained from sound research is transformed into clinical practice, leading to medical practice that is evidence-based. An important feature of the research is that it is a continuous process that leads to more questions at the end of it.

Though the research question has been described later but it would be important to review some of the features of research questions here (*see* below).

Before framing a proper research question one should *introspect a lot as they pertain to specific discipline or assignment. Additionally, one should consider items on the research list. One should jot down everything one knows about the topic as quickly as one can. Research questions should be able to find out the possible "gaps" in the existing knowledge.* It is important to know that the open-ended questions often lead to good a research question. The questions asked before the research starts should have the following properties (Table 1.1).

Table. 1.1: General properties of research question

- *Clear and precisely stated*
- Not too broad, nor is it too narrow
- Open-ended, as opposed to closed

HOW TO FRAME A RESEARCH QUESTION?

Though the process has been detailed later in the text but often, we do not know what we are curious about until we read about subjects that interest us first in details. Going to the library, and search online academic and professional sites related to discipline of interests and topics can give us more clarity.

Science

Science is a "body of established knowledge through the observation, identification, investigation, and theoretical explanation of natural phenomenon". Usually the ultimate goal of science is the theory generation and verification by using research methods.

Theory

This is a set of interrelated constructs and propositions that specify relations among variables to explain and predict phenomena. It should be simple, consistent with observed relationships, tentative and verifiable by research methods.

Research Methods/Methodology

Research methodology is the way/s one *collects and analyzes data.* These are the methods developed for acquiring trustworthy knowledge via reliable and valid procedures. Research should have certain characters (Table 1.2). The process is best learnt via practice (Fig. 1.2).

Table 1.2: Features of research

- Objective-scientifically sound
- Precise-accurate
- Verifiable-testable
- Parsimonious-should save, time and money
- Empirical-learnt by experience
- Logical-factual
- Probabilistic-explained by rules of probability

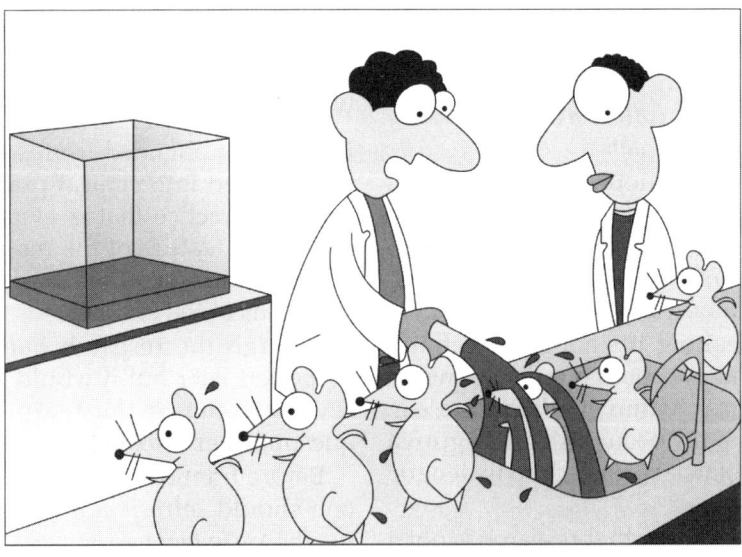

Fig. 1.2: Research is a process, which is best learnt by doing rather than by didactic lectures

Type of Research

Research could be of several types: grossly, in medicine, there are three types of researches.

- Descriptive, e.g. what percentage of dementia patients smoke? What percentage of diabetic patients do not follow regular dietary advice?
  - *Performed by*: Cross sectional study.
- Relational (associational), e.g. link between age and exercise; brain functions and nutritional, etc.
  - *Performed by*: Case-control study.
- Causal, e.g. effect of behavior change intervention on exercise participation; lung cancer and smoking, etc.
  - *Performed by*: Cohort study.

Scientific method: Scientific involves the principles and processes regarded as characteristic of or necessary for scientific investigation. Process or approach to generating valid and trustworthy knowledge (Fig. 1.3).

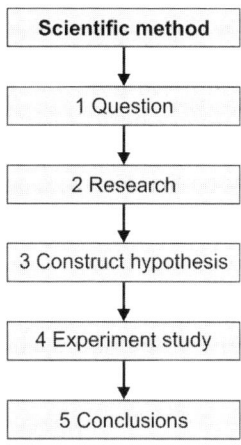

Fig. 1.3: The process of research is best learnt by scientific methods

Francis Galton

Francis Galton was a British inventor and sociologist with a deep interest in scientific method. He was of the view that science should be learnt via observations → data collection → analysis and interpretation →

theory generation. Several features of the scientific methods are given below (Table 1.3):

Table 1.3: Steps followed in scientific methods

1. Choose a question to investigate
2. Identify a hypothesis related to the question
3. Make testable predictions in the hypothesis
4. Design an experiment to answer hypothesis question
5. Collect data in experiment
6. Determine results and assess their validity
7. Determine if results support or refute your hypothesis

Basic elements of scientific methods

- *Empiricism*: The notion that enquiry is conducted through observation and knowledge verified through evidence that either comes via experience or has come via testing of facts experimentally. The latter is more important than former in medicine.

- *Determinism*: The notion that events occur according to regular laws and causes. The goal of research is to discover these governing.

- *Skepticism*: The notion that any proposition is open to analysis and critique.

These features should lead us to form a research question (Tables 1.1 and 1.2).

1. **High index of suspicion:** Suspicion that a factor (exposure) may influence occurrence of disease or a noted health outcome.
   - Observations in clinical practice
   - Examination of disease/outcome patterns
     - Do subpopulations have higher or lower rates?
     - Are disease rates increased in the presence of certain factors?

- Observations in laboratory research
- Theoretical speculation

2. **Identifying variable:** Identify variables you are interested in:
   - Exposure—risk factor, protective factor, predictor variable, treatment.
   - Outcome—disease, event.

3. **Form a hypothesis:** Formulate a specific hypothesis is an important step:
   - Frame a hypothesis which seeks to answer a specific question about the relationship between an exposure and an outcome.

All kind of research starts with an idea that may come from the professional experience, burning questions, literature, professional meetings, and discussions. That can lead us to the research questions (Table 1.4).

Table 1.4: Properties of a research question (FINER)

- Feasible
- Interesting
- Novel
- Ethical
- Relevant

Feasibility

- **Feasible**
  - *Subjects*: Healthy, diseased or both
  - *Resources*: What kind needed?
  - *Manageable*: Look for feasibility
  - *Data*: Primary or secondary

Scientific Interest

The Topic Should be Interesting

Novelty

- **Novel**
  - In relation to previous findings
    - Confirm or refute?
  - New setting, new population
- **Ethical**
  - Social or scientific value
  - Safe

Relevance

- **Relevant**
  - Advance scientific knowledge?
  - Influence clinical practice?
  - Impact health policy?
  - Guide future research?

Variable

A variable is "any property of a person, thing, event, setting, and so on that is not fixed." Variable is any observation that can take on different values. For example, age, sex, weight, height, blood pressure, heart rate, etc.

- **Is one variable related to another?**
  - "Is X related to Y? What is the effect of X on Y?", etc.

Dependent and Independent Variable

The variable determines, influences, or produces the change in the other main variable is called independent variable. The other variable is usually the dependent variable or the subject variable. This variable is dependent on or influenced by the independent variable(s).

Independent variable has a presumed effect on the dependent variable and can influence the outcome. May or may not be manipulated. Dependent variable on the other hand is something that varies with a change in the independent variable. It is hence, *also called outcome* variable.

Attribute

This is a specific value of a variable.

Variable	Attribute
Age	19, 20, 21, 25, etc.
Gender	Males or females

Bibliography

1. Bos JM, van den Bemt PM, De Smet PA, Kramers C. The effect of prescriber education on medication related patient harm in the hospital: a systematic review. Br J Clin Pharmacol. 2016 Dec 5. doi: 10.1111/bcp.13200. [Epub ahead of print].

2. Canova C, Pitter G, Schifano P. [A systematic review of epidemiological cohort studies based on the Italian Medical Birth Register. Is it time to think of a multicentric birth cohort?] Epidemiol Prev. 2016 Nov-Dec; 40(6): 439–452. Review. Italian.

3. Dias S, Welton NJ, Sutton AJ, Ades AE. Introduction to Evidence Synthesis for Decision Making [Internet]. London: National Institute for Health and Care Excellence (NICE); 2012 Apr.

Research Question

WHAT IS A RESEARCH QUESTION?

The research question is the starting point of the study. Everything in medical research starts from the research question. It will determine the population to be studied, the setting for the study, the data to be collected, and the time period for the study and many more things. A clear and concisely stated research question is the most important requirement for a successful study.

FRAMING A RESEARCH QUESTION (Fig. 2.1)

Researchers must, first, pose a question that narrows down the 'topic' to a single problem (and often to a hypothesis). It should have following characteristics (Table 2.1):

Table 2.1: Features of a research questions
- Is not too big and not too small
- Grounded (as in simple)
- Builds on what is known
- Promises some new knowledge
- Will 'last' the duration of the research
- Practical and doable
- Looks for something new
- Always relevant

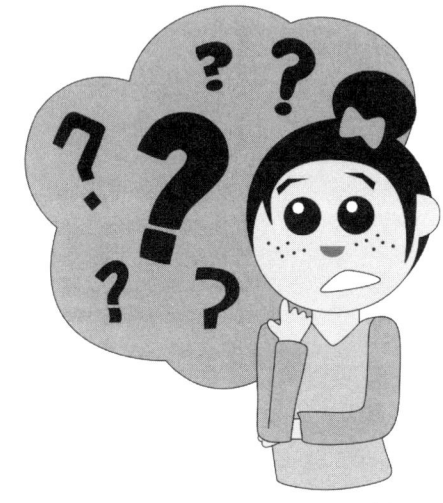

Fig. 2.1: Research question is beginning of the scientific process

It is generally said that if one does not get the research question right at the start of the PhD; one would probably not enjoy the studies and the chance of successful outcome would be reduce. It is however important to know that it should not be of a tall order and that sets frustratingly difficult expectations which are difficult to follow, i.e. it should be reasonable, and feasible.

Especially in the PhD level research, the formulation of research questions helps assessors judge whether the candidate has presented an original, integrated argument, and the significance of that contribution could be analyzed.

Even though research questions will have evolved in the beginning but the final work/paper/thesis should demonstrate the research question and its value in adding knowledge and understanding.

LEVELS OF RESEARCH QUESTIONS

Research question refers to the precise focus of original and independent research that leads to useful *findings*. Subsidiary questions guide the *operational stages* of the inquiry, the steps as one builds the answer and *address assumptions by doing experiments.*

A higher-level question shows the more general class of knowledge that the research could contribute: It is the essence of the question, and could be the reason for investigation. It actually is the *significance of findings.*

PROCESS OF GENERATING A RESEARCH QUESTION

The most important prerequisite for this research is a well-cultivated curiosity. This seems to be a common characteristic possessed by notable researchers. Beyond being curious, these individuals also had the patience and tenacity to follow a question until satisfied with the answer.

TIPS TO GENERATE A GOOD RESEARCH QUESTION

Though formulating a research is a tedious task, but still some useful tips could be given to ensure formulation of a good research question (Table 2.2).

STEPS IN FORMULATING RESEARCH QUESTIONS

Formulating a research question starts with an idea. However, it has to be backed by

Table 2.2: Useful tips to form a research question

- Careful observations
- Look at draft of research question/hypothesis
- Application of new technology
- Based upon experience
- Scientific communications
- Skeptical attitude
- Question validity of commonly held beliefs
- Revise and rewrite

practical methods and methods (Table 2.3). A good research question should be able to study the variables under considerations, the population being studied and the testability of the question.

Table 2.3: Formulating a research question

- Generate on idea
- Identify a question
- Modify the question
- Form a hypothesis

Remembering Attributes

There are several features that a good research question encompasses (*see* acronym below). FINER is a widely used criteria.

FINER Criteria for Suitability of Research Question

- **Feasible**
  - Adequate numbers of subjects?
  - Adequate technical expertise?
  - Affordable in time and money?
  - Is it possible to measure or manipulate the variables?
- **Interesting**
  - To the investigator/sponsor?
- **Novel**
  - To the field/to the audience?
- **Ethical**
  - Potential harm to subjects?
  - Potential breech of subject confidentiality?
- **Relevant**
  - To scientific knowledge/theory?
  - To organizational, health or social management and policy?
  - To individual welfare?

Bibliography

1. Blaikie, N. (2000). Designing social research.
2. Examples derived from studies designed by Di Buchan (skilled migrants) and Marsden award winners: JE Reese (stories); B Thompson

(old brains); H Petrie (slavery); CH Brown, Grattan (hormones); MK Savage (volcanoes) (www. marsden.rsnz.org).

3. Hawke, G. (2010). Presentation to School of Government PhD students.

4. Postgraduate thesis and forming research question. http://www.brighthub.com/ education/postgraduate/articles/68825. aspx (Accessed online dated 9th December 2016).

5. Properties of a good research question. http://universalteacher.com/1/characteristics-of-a-good-research-question/ (Accessed online dated May 22nd 2017).

Research Process

Learning objectives

Purpose of research could be gaining some familiarity with a topic, discovering some of its main dimensions, and possibly planning more structured research or discovering new facts/technologies, etc. Alternatively, it may also be describing a phenomena or a topic also. It is important to know that research should represent some significant addition to our knowledge. This has to follow a particular process.

Research Process

Process of research starts with the development of a question that has been formed before hand or that has been motivated by experience. One should state the question as a testable hypothesis. Remember, if you cannot do it, you still do not have a good question. It starts with the searching the literature to see if the question has been answered totally or partially. It flows systematically (Table 3.1). In general, a research design is like a blueprint for the research. Research methodology concerns how the design is implemented, how the research is carried out (Fig. 3.1).

Research is not just about the collection of data. Data collection is important, but it is simply part of a wider process—the *research process*.

Table 3.1: Steps involved in research process

- Problem definition
- Literature review
- Selection of research design, subjects, and data collection techniques
- Data gathering
- Data processing and analysis
- Implications, conclusions, and recommendations

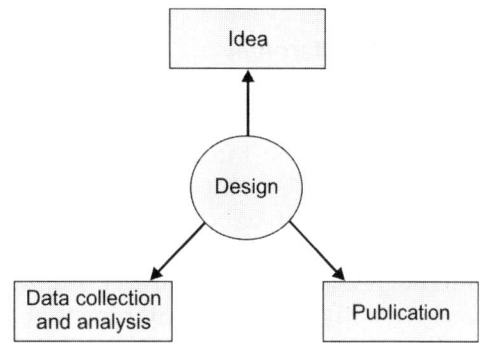

Fig. 3.1: Publication is the essence of science but follows a conceptual framework before the results get published. It is noted that scientific research involves a systematic proves that focuses on being objective and gathering information for analysis so that it can lead to logical conclusion. The scientific process is a multi-step process where the steps are linked with other steps

The research process follows several steps, e.g. selection of topic, reviewing the literature, developing theoretical and conceptual frameworks, clarifying research question, developing a research design, collecting data, analysing data, and drawing conclusions, etc.

Relating the research question to the research process will allow one to develop and answer research question in a logical and systematic manner.

Problem Identification

The problem must be clearly recognized and one should determine information already available and what further information is required, as well as the best approach for obtaining it. Additionally, one should obtain and assess information objectively to help take the informed the decision.

One should be able to describe the broader context or the background of the problem. Also, state the objectives or purposes clearly. One should not forget to inform reader about the scope of the study, including defining any terms, limitations, or restrictions, etc. one has to state the hypothesis clearly. This is a crucial stage, as an inappropriate topic or question will often lead to irretrievable difficulties later in the research.

Review of the Literature

A literature review essentially consists of critically reading, evaluating and organising existing literature on the topic to assess the state of knowledge in the area. During this stage one should aim to become an 'expert' in the chosen field of research. This happens only after through search. That means, it should be exhaustive without leaving anything that has been done.

Review of literature helps giving the theoretical rationale of problem being studied, i.e. what research has been done and how it relates to the problem under study. It is also helpful to divide the literature into subtopics for ease of reading. It is important to focus on the quality of literature. One should be sure to include leading scientists in the research area. These individuals are usually the opinion makers and drive the direction of research for decades.

Research Question

Initial research questions are chosen, investigated and often rejected for a number of reasons, e.g. the question may lack sufficient focus or the conceptual framework has not identified problems clearly. Also, there may be too many moderating or intervening variables. Additionally, the project may be unfeasible in terms of complexity, access, facilities or resources. For details of research question, readers may go through Chapter 2.

As one reads the literature, one should be continually developing and refining theoretical

and conceptual frameworks. Theoretical framework refers to the underlying theoretical approach that one would adopt to underpin the study. The conceptual framework defines and organises the concepts important within the study.

Research Design (Fig. 3.2)

The research design indicates the steps that will need to be take and the sequence they will occur. Each design can rely on one more data collection techniques, e.g. case-control, cross sectional studies. They may help in assess reliability and validity of the methods used. Critical consideration in determining methodology is the selection of subjects as the next step.

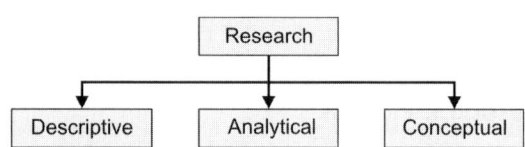

Fig. 3.2: Broadly research can be descriptive, analytical or conceptual. The latter is used in psychosocial sciences

Research designs answer some of the common questions like:

- What data is needed to collect to answer this question?

- What is the best way to collect this data?

- What overall research design should be used? For example, a cross-sectional, experimental or longitudinal design, etc.

- Will the data need to be primary or secondary data?

- What methods, e.g. interviews, questionnaire surveys and so on, will be best to collect the primary data?

- Who should participate in the research?

- What are the exact procedures that one should adopt in data collection to ensure reliability and validity?

- Are there any ethical issues associated with the research?

One should determine what tools, materials, personnel, time, and so forth are necessary to obtain and analyzed the data based on your reading of the literature. Feasibility is very important and an important question that should come to the investigator's mind is that: Given the requirements, is the study feasible? Additionally, one may need to revise the question and hypothesis and/or alter the variables according to resources and time available.

Choosing the subjects: One would have to choose the appropriate subjects including controls, if appropriate from whom data on the variables can be obtained.

Case definitions: A clinical case definition or simply a case definition deals with the clinical criteria that the instigator must find first. This should be easy, comprehensible and usable by all.

Variables under study should first be first defined by *conceptual definitions* that explain the concept the variable is trying to capture. Later, variables should be defined by operational definitions which are definitions for how variable will be measured. For example, hypertension and diabetes should be defined in a workable manner if they are included in the study.

Revision: One should revise the question and hypothesis based on the review of the literature if needed. Research question may also need to be revised, based upon the hypothesis, and variables to match the subjects to whom one may have access.

Statistician: One should discuss the proposed study with a biostatistician or some experienced epidemiologist in clinical research before starting the project. After the data collection has already started it becomes not only difficult or at times it may seem to be "trying to revive the dead".

Pilot studies: A pilot study or also called pilot project is a small scale study done to know about the feasibility, time, cost, possible adverse events, etc. one of the most important feature of such a study when done for quantitative data is that it can provide effect size. This is very helpful in calculation of sample size for the studies.

If not much is known about the topic and its parameters, one must pretest. This is called pilot study. One should design the sampling schemes and the questionnaires should be coded if it is used.

Data collection: Data collection should be started after the ethical approval of the project has been obtained. Unfortunately, many novices begin this step too soon thereby compromising the study's worth. See everything has its own value: ethical issues need handling and respected too.

Data analysis: Preferably, one should analyze the data, with the help of a biostatistician. However if one is confident, one can do it alone too. Initially, one should describe demographics of the data. One should choose appropriate statistical techniques and always look for patterns in data. "Milk the data dry" is a useful expression where the data can be analyzed from all angles.

Interpretation of data: Make sure to consider the audience for which the research has been done. One should discuss implications for the population of interest and future research in the area. That proves the dictum that "research begins with a question and ends with a question".

Concluding: Conclusions should relate back to the focused research question that was formulated in the beginning. One quick way of checking the same is to look at the title of the paper and tile and conclusion should match. One can evaluate how successful one has been in achieving research objectives, and highlight the strengths and weaknesses of the research. One should always do recommendations for further research in case the conclusion is such.

Writing a report/publication: Write it up for publication is the essence of science. This is what separates the academic from the nonacademic clinical researchers. After the paper is accepted (which might take several attempts), one can analyze if it is making some sense. Attempt should be done to publish in same/related area. Selection of the proper journal is the key in this regard.

Bibliography

1. Basic steps in research. http://www.nhcc.edu/student-resources/library/doinglibraryresearch/basic-steps-in-the-research-process (Downloaded on May 6th 2017).

2. Research methodology. https://olinuris.library.cornell.edu/content/seven-steps-research-process (Downloaded on May 6th 2017).

3. Steps of research. https://olinuris.library.cornell.edu/content/seven-steps-research-process (Downloaded on May 6th 2017).

Association in Medical Research

Learning objectives

Exploring associations is one of the major aims of doing medical research. There are two main kinds of variables: qualitative and quantitative and there are several types of tests that can check association between these. Correlations, chi-square, and linear and multiple regression are main methods of checking associations between variables.

Univariate Verses Bivariate Variables

Before understanding association it is important to know that we need to consider at least two variables for studying association, e.g. height and weight, sun exposure and vitamin D levels and eating fatty food and dyslipidemia, etc. These are typical examples of *bivariate* relationships.

It is often the case that one may wish to move to examine the relationships between several variables; called *multivariate* analysis.

In multivariate analysis, several independent or predictors variables are studied with multiple outcome or dependent variables. This study is done using matrix algebra and most of the multivariate analyses are correlational in nature.

So basically, multivariate analysis uses data that arises from more than one variable. Multivariate analysis may be close to reality where the variables may be interrelated.

Apart from correlation, multivariate regression may be performed by a technique that estimates a single regression model with one than one outcome variable. When there is more than one predictor model; model is called multiple regression models. Usually, the dependent and independent variables are one each in the study; however, in factorial design, there may be more than one independent variable.

Association

It is important to explore what kind of relationship exists between the variables (Fig. 4.1). From the results of the study, one should be able to assess if the statistical relationship exists between two or more events, characteristics, or other variables. Additionally, one may see if there is a statistical relationship, or association, between exposure and disease/outcome? (Fig. 4.1).

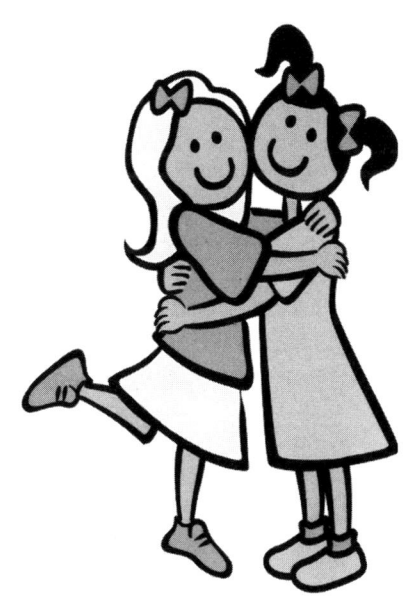

Fig. 4.1: Exploring association is one of major aims of biomedical research

One should be able to see if:
- There is no relationship
- Positive relationship exists
- Negative relationship is there
- Curvilinear relationship is present.

Probing Associations

Chi-square test, paired t-test, correlation and regression analysis are commonly used to probe the associations between variables.

Measuring Associations

Associations are usually scaled between zero to 1; 1 being perfect relationship while zero means no association. It can be positive or negative. Tests of significance are sometimes used to measure associations and start with the assumption that there are no associations (zero) and this is taken to be the null hypothesis. If the observed value of measured association is different from zero, the alternative hypothesis is accepted (Fig. 4.2).

Statistical Association

Statistical association deals with the degree to which the rate of disease or outcome in persons with a specific exposure is either higher or lower than the rate of disease or outcome among those without that exposure.

Hypothesis is a specific statement of prediction and is of two main types: alternative *vs* null and it can also be one-tailed or two-tailed.

Chi-Squared Tests

Chi-square test of independence is a very easy way to find out if there is association between two variables. It can also tell about the size of this association. A cross classification table can be used to obtain expected number of cases under the assumption of no relationship among the variables. Then the value of chi-square statistic can tell about if there is any association between variables in cross classification table. Nature of association however cannot be tested by this. Additionally, it is difficult to assume what change in one variable can bring when other is changed. Though the chi-squared test statistic will indicate if there is association that excites between variables but it cannot tell a lot about this.

The Pearson chi-square test is used to test whether a statistically significant relationship exists between two categorical variables (e.g. gender and type of car). It accompanies a cross tabulation between the two variables. Categorical independent and dependent variable needed.

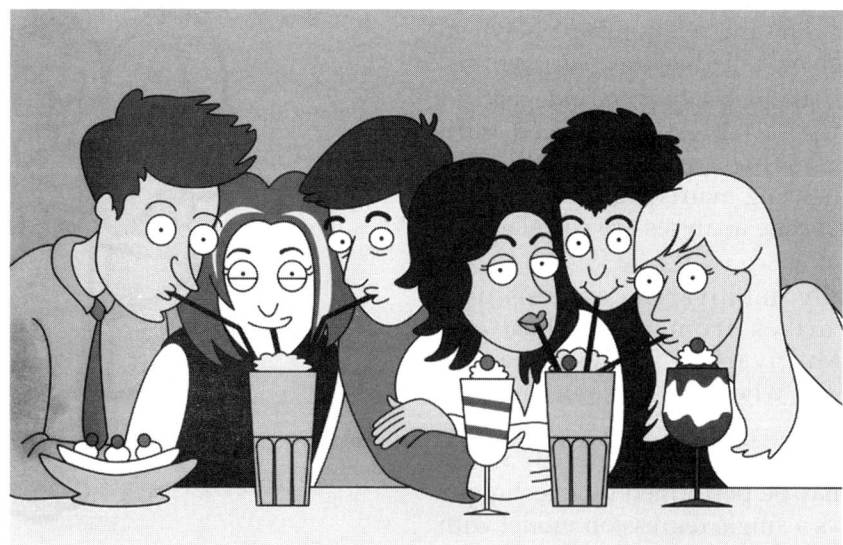

Fig. 4.2: Associations can be strong or weak, positive or negative and can be graded from 0–1

Correlation

Correlation tests (Pearson correlation) are used to examine relationships between two or more quantitative/numerical variables. Correlation tests also measure the strength and direction of a relationship between variables (Fig. 4.3).

One should ask like how many variables are present and which one is the independent variable, and which one is the dependent variable? What types of variables are they? So is the correlation appropriate or not? (Fig. 4.3).

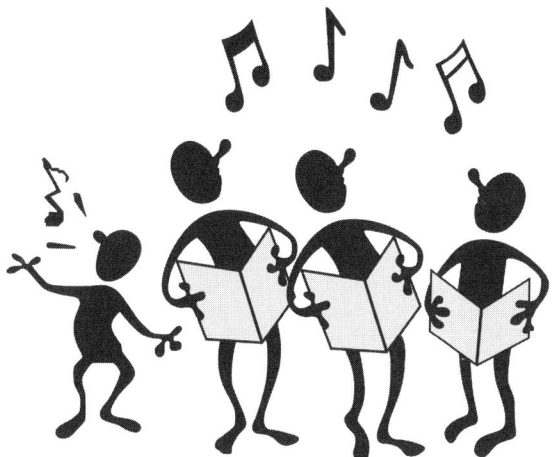

Fig. 4.3: Out of the wild array of data, the correlation analysis can show if the relationship exists or not

A positive correlation between height and age means that higher values on the height variable (e.g. taller people) are associated with higher values on the age variable (e.g. older people).

A negative correlation means that higher values on the height variable (e.g. taller people) are associated with lower values on age variable (e.g. younger people). The *p-values* tells whether the relationship or correlation between the variables are statistically significant ($p < .05$).

Strength of Correlation

Correlations have different strengths and is measured in terms of correlation coefficient (r):

0.10 to 0.29	Weak correlation
0.30 to 0.49	Moderate correlation
0.5 and above	Strong correlation

Regression Analysis

Regression analyses are used to examine the effect of different (predictor/independent) variables on a single outcome (dependent) variable (Fig. 4.3). The use of the term "prediction" is central to regression analyses. One examines whether if one variable predicts (explains/impacts) another variable.

The independent or predictor variables must be either dichotomous (categorical variable with only 2 categories/groups) or quantitative/numerical variables. The dependent variable must be a quantitative/numerical variable. Simple linear regression examines the relationship between one predictor variable and one outcome variable. It is noteworthy that it produces the same results as a bivariate Pearson correlation.

Multiple regression is a more popular extension of linear regression. Multiple regression examines the effects of the multiple predictors or independent variables on a single outcome variable. The output is same as the linear regression analysis, and so is the interpretation (Fig. 4.4).

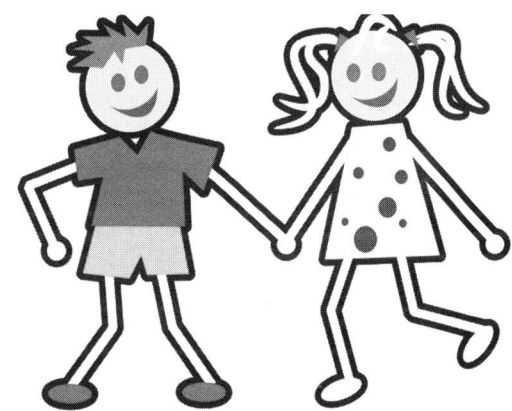

Fig. 4.4: Correlation can just tell about the presence of association but regression can tell about causality

Assessing Validity of Association

The foremost question is to see if there does exist the observed association? (Fig. 4.5).

One should then try to see if the association between variables is valid or not? Also, one should see if there are there alternative

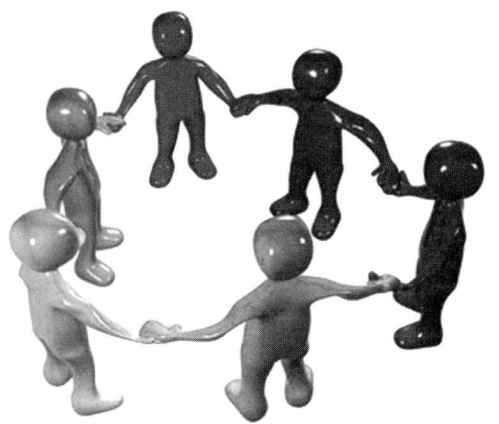

Fig. 4.5: Associations in biomedical sciences are core of several types of research. The association between variables should however be a valid one

explanations for the association? Has it arisen by chance or bias or confounding, etc.

Bibliography

1. Berry KJ, Mielke PW. A family of multivariate measures of association for nominal independent variables. Educational and Psychological Measurement, 1992;52(1): 41–55.

2. Cohen J, Nee JC. Estimators for two measures of association for set correlation. Educational and Psychological Measurement. 1984;44(4): 907–917.

3. Measuring association. http://www. statisticssolutions.com/directory-of-statistical-analyses-correlation-measures-of-association/ (Assessed online on 2nd May 2017).

Research Hypothesis

Learning objectives

Broadly speaking, hypothesis is an educated guess that can be statistically tested. Hypotheses provides prediction about the relationship among two or more variables or groups based on a theory or the previous research. Hypotheses are assumptions or theories that a researcher makes and eventually tests. Hypothesis is the spine of medical research. A test of hypothesis is a statistical test that can be used to know if there was enough evidence in the data sample collected to infer that a certain situation is true for entire population or not. A hypothesis test always examines two hypotheses about the population (the null and the alternative hypothesis). Based on the sample data, the acceptance or rejection of null hypothesis is done.

Table 5.1: Characteristics of research hypothesis

- Identifies the predicted relationship between two or more variables
- Tells about testability
- Based on sound scientific theory/rationale
- Clear and understandable
- Measurable
- Contain independent and dependent variable

Table 5.2: Types of hypothesis

- Null
- Alternative
- Directional
- Other

HYPOTHESIS

Hypothesis is a statement about the relationship between two or more variables. Hypothesis converts the question into a statement that predicts an expected outcome. It is considered to be a unit or subset of the research problem. One would have to set up an experiment or situation to test. Hypothesis suggest relationships (or lack thereof) between and among variables. It can also predict causes and relationships prior to testing. It may have several characteristics (Table 5.1). Types of hypothesis are given in Table 5.2.

Characters of Hypothesis (Table 5.1)

A hypothesis can direct observations and identifies the variables examined and helps specifying the data to be collected. It also helps describing relationship among variables, which is a major aim of medical research. Additionally, a hypothesis can state that as one

variable increases, the other will decrease; as one variables increases, the other will increase, and so on. Most important utility of the hypothesis is that the results of a sample will translate to a population (external validity).

Hypotheses can estimate population characteristics by studying a *small sample*. Correlating various variables will give dimensions to the research data. Hypothesis can allow the outlining of the differences among two or more populations. A clearly laid hypothesis can show the possible cause and effect; which is the ultimate aim of many medical researchers.

Depicting Hypothesis

A hypothesis in statistical calculations is depicted by Greek symbols. For example, if M = mean, then μ (mu: mew) = *population mean*. Roman Letters (e.g. A, B, C, D) can be used to represent statistics.

Greek letters (e.g. α, β) are used to represent parameters.

Alpha (α) is the significance level; probability of committing a Type 1 Error (α = 0.05). In other words, p = probability value (p = 0.05).

Null hypothesis = (H_0: $\mu_1 - \mu_2 = 0$ or H_0: $\mu_1 = \mu_2$) and the alternative hypothesis = (H_1: $\mu_1 - \mu_2 \neq 0$ or H_1: $\mu_1 \neq \mu_2$). Alternative hypothesis is also depicted as H_A.

Types of Hypothesis

It can be of several types, but broadly of two types:

a. **Research hypothesis:** This is a statement of the relationship among two or more variables or groups. The acceptance or rejection of a research hypothesis is based on resolving a logical alternative with a null hypothesis. For example, graduate students who read the text in research methodology will score higher in Msc/MD/PhD entrance examination than students who did not read their research methodology book.

Research hypotheses can be stated as *directional* or *nondirectional*. Directional hypotheses predict the specific relationship among two or more variables or groups:

$$H_0: \mu_1 \leq \mu_2 \quad H_1: \mu_1 > \mu_2$$

Directional hypothesis specifies the direction of the relationship between independent and dependent variables.

Nondirectional hypotheses predict that there will be differences among two or more groups, but *do not specify the direction of the differences.*

$$H_0: \mu_1 = \mu_2 \quad H_1: \mu_1 \neq \mu_2$$

Nondirectional hypothesis shows the existence of a relationship between variables but no direction is specified.

b. **Statistical hypothesis:** Statistical Hypotheses are mathematical, or logical statements that help researchers interpret the results of the research. Statistical hypotheses consist of the null hypothesis (H_0), the hypothesis of no difference and the

alternative hypothesis (H_1 or H_A) which is similar in form to the research hypothesis.
Null: (H_0: $\mu_1 - \mu_2 = 0$)
Alternative: (H_1: $\mu_1 - \mu_2 \neq 0$)

Null hypothesis: The absence of a relationship or difference in the results; any relationship or difference is due to chance or sampling error. For example, there will be no difference in the comprehensive test scores of students who read the text in research methodology and those who did not read their research methodology book.

Alternative: Alternative hypothesis expresses a relationship between the variables under study. It points a direction and requires "assumption" that is specified and objective.

Students who read the book of research methodology will score higher on their comprehensive exams than graduate students who did not read their research methods text.

The null hypothesis always implies that there is no relation or statistical difference between variables or groups while the alternative hypothesis implies that there is a meaningful relationship among variables or groups.

A clearly formed hypothesis is the key to success. It should have several characteristics (Table 5.3).

Hypothesis Testing

After formulating a hypothesis; frame the hypothesis in a format that is testable, i.e. develop it a study design. Finally, one is expected to test the hypothesis.

Table 5.3: Characteristics of good hypothesis

- Constructs are clear
- Relationship (sign, direction if experimental, type of moderation) is clear
- Population often included
- Design/statistical method often clear
- Mean differences clear
- Comparison specified

The hypothesis formed during the study may be support, not supported, or rejection.

* *Hypothesis testing is a four phase procedure*:
  - Phase I: Research hypotheses, design, and variables
  - Phase II: Statistical hypotheses
  - Phase III: Hypotheses testing
  - Phase IV: Decision/interpretation

a. *Hypothesis design*: One has to begin by stating the hypothesis for research. After this, one will have to decide on a research design based on the research problem, hypotheses, and what would really want to be able to say about the results (e.g. if one wants to say that A caused B, one will need an experimental or time-series design; if probable cause is sufficient, a quasi-experimental design would be appropriate). It is very important to operationally define your variables.

For example, if we are taking diabetes then an operational definition of diabetes will be needed. Likewise, hypertension will have to be clearly defined as well. Recall that one variable can have more than one operational definition.

b. *Statistical hypothesis*: This is a critical step where one would have to analyze the chosen statistical procedures. One will have to write one statistical null hypotheses for each operational definition of each variable that reflects that statistical operations to be performed. For example, presence of diabetes contributes to dementia or it does not contribute.

c. *Hypothesis testing*: Complete the following steps for each statistical null hypothesis: Select a significance level (alpha) and compute the value of the test statistic (e.g. F, r, t).

One will have to compare the obtained value of the test statistics with the critical value associated with the selected significance level or compare the obtained *p-value* with the pre-selected alpha value. If the obtained value of the test statistic is greater than the critical value (or if the obtained *p-value* is less than the pre-selected alpha value), reject the null hypothesis. If the obtained value is less than the critical value of the test hypothesis, fail to reject the null hypothesis. Another way of looking it is that if the *p-value* is less than or equal to alpha, reject the null hypothesis.

d. *Decision*: For each research hypothesis, consider the decisions regarding the statistical null hypotheses. One would have to cautiously explain the findings with respect to the research hypotheses. It is important to list and discuss the limitations of the study. Factors that could threat the validity of the study should be taken into account as well. It is generally recommended that one reports the effect size along with the value of the test statistic and the *p-value*. An alternative is to report confidence intervals.

Several questions need to be answered before final decision about accepting or rejecting the null hypothesis is taken. For example, is it possible that the observations in the study could have occurred by chance? We use a variety of statistical procedures to test null hypotheses. The choice of which procedure we use depends on a variety of factors including: the research hypothesis, data, sampling strategy, and what we want to be able to say as a result of our testing.

In order to test a hypothesis, we compare the obtained value of a test statistic (e.g. the obtained F) to a critical value of the test statistic (e.g. a critical F; also called table value) that is associated with the preset significance level (alpha). There are several statistical tools to do the same (Table 5.1).

If the obtained value of the test statistic is greater than the critical value, we determine that there is a significant difference or relationship. The test statistic could be the specific statistic (i.e. the tool) that is chosen to test the null hypothesis, e.g. F (ANOVA), t (student t test), r (correlation coefficient).

Calculated value is the actual value obtained when applying the test statistic to the collected data. The probability value associated with the obtained value is *p-value*. Critical value is the critical value (also called table value) of the test statistic that is associated with the chosen significance level (alpha). Note that if the obtained value is greater that the critical value, the result is considered to be significant. Statistical procedures that are commonly used for hypothesis testing are given below (Table 5.4):

Table 5.4: Statistical tests of hypothesis testing

Correlation

Analysis of variance (ANOVA)

Analysis of covariance (ANCOVA)

Regression

Multivariate analysis of variance (MANOVA)

Student t-tests

Chi-square test: Each of these procedures has an associated test statistic, which is used to determine significance. For example, ANOVA, ANCOVA, and regression use F statistics and their associated *p-values*. Multivariate procedures, like MANOVA, use a variety of test statistics with interesting names, like Wilk's lambda. These are then related to a more common test statistic, like F. All test statistics are eventually related to a probability distribution and a *p-value*. These *p-values* mean the same thing across test statistics.

Errors in Hypothesis Testing

In hypothesis testing, one must be comfortable with two types of errors: Type 1 and 2. In general, the errors are mistakes that we can make when judging the null hypothesis (Tables 5.5 and 5.6).

Type 1 Error

Type 1 error is what happens when the tested hypothesis is falsely rejected. (It is when you we say we found something, but that

Table 5.5: Error decision chart

Decision	H_0 true	H_1 true
Reject H_0	Type 1 error	Correct (1β)
Fail to reject	Correct (1α)	Type 2 β

Table 5.6: Factors related to study power

Sample size

Effect size

Study design

Significance level

something is really an error!). It is like saying "rope is a snake" and be convinced about it as well. It is actually the probability of committing an error when accepting or rejecting a hypothesis. Since, this could lead to introduction of a drug in case the hypothesis testing involves the drug; hence a *type 1 error* is a false positive.

Type 2 Error

Type 2 error is happens when a false tested hypothesis is not rejected. That is, the difference was there but we were unable to spot it. Hence, a *type 2 error* is a false negative. Alpha is the level of probability (pre-set by the researcher) that the tested hypothesis will be falsely rejected.

Alpha is the pre-set risk of a *type 1 error*. In other words, alpha is the degree of risk that you accept, in advance of conducting the study, that what you find will be an error. Beta is the probability that a false null hypothesis will not be rejected. Beta is the probability that you will not find what you are looking for if, in fact, it is really there. Error decision chart is given in Table 5.5.

Study Power

Power of the study is "the probability of rejecting a null hypothesis that is, in fact, false" (Table 5.6).

Cohen defines statistical power is a function of "the preset significance criterion (alpha), the reliability of sample results, and the effect size (the actual size) of the difference or strength of the relationship".

Put simply, statistical power is the pro-bability of finding relationships or differences that in fact exist. This is the major tool that "empowers" the scientist to be able to spot the difference between the groups.

In terms of beta, the probability of a type 2 error is statistical power, i.e. $= 1 - beta$. So, if a study has a 20% chance of being negative, even though the study has been done and the difference is there, the statistical power of the study is: $1-0.10 = 0.80$.

Alpha and beta errors are directly, but not perfectly related. Considering complex interrelationships of the above criteria, one can say that the researcher can easily set alpha, but cannot easily set beta. Lowering alpha increases beta and lowers the power. Increasing alpha decreases beta and increases power. Power of the study is affected by several factors (Table 5.3).

Effect Size

Effect size refers to the amount of common variance between the independent variable/s and the dependent variable/s, or the degree to which changes in the independent variable/s results in changes in the dependent/s. For example, if we were to know the difference in weight of two groups of students who study in two different colleges; then we could compare the two. Now to be able to consider it a significant difference we have to keep a limit. A few grams cannot be the effect size; however a few kilograms can be.

Significance Level

This is also called probability value: The probability that observed relationships or differences are due to chance. This is denoted by Greek letter α (Alpha) and is also known as significance level or rejection region. It is the level of probability set by the researcher as grounds for rejection of the null hypothesis. 1 Alpha is the probability level associated with the critical value of the test statistic.

What happens when the obtained probability (p) is less than our predetermined alpha? The results are considered to be significant. The significance also occurs when the obtained value of the test statistic is greater than the critical value of the test statistic.

Alpha Inflation

Multiple comparisons can increase alpha, the probability of a *type 1 error*. For example, doing repeated t-tests in case with multiple groups is unreliable. That is why in such a situations, statisticians choose ANOVA rather than repeated paired t-tests. The probability of a *type 1 error* escalates with the number of comparisons made in such a study.

Another way to guard against alpha inflation is to use a Bonneferoni-type procedure and to split alpha by the number of comparisons. There are a variety of such procedures that can be used according to the relative importance of the tested hypotheses.

The problem with reducing alpha is that it inflates beta. In situations in which alpha inflation is accepted due to a problem with power, one must look to replications for confidence in the findings.

Generate Hypothesis

Generating a hypothesis starts with a research question. For example, the research question can be is the frequency of diabetes higher in cases with dementias? Now, it can be higher or lower or same. So the hypothesis can be

- H_0: Frequency of diabetes in dementias is not same as that of age matched controls.
- H_1: Frequency of diabetes in dementias is same as that of age matched controls.

It is very important to know that hypotheses should be developed before data are collected. Calculation of study sample size, what issues should be involved in data collection, etc. should be sorted well in advance. It should be followed by the proper analysis of the data and data interpretation.

How to Form Hypothesis?

Forming hypothesis is based upon the research question. Observations from literature (students generally PubMed or www.google.com or www.googlescholar.com), natural experiments (e.g. post-traumatic stress disorders in war torn zones), multinational comparisons (e.g. happiness indices of various countries) could be helpful to form hypotheses. Additionally, descriptive studies (assessment of person, place, and time characteristics) or creativity/ innovation indices of different nations could be helpful to form the hypothesis. It can be expressed in two forms:

H_0: "Null" hypothesis (assumed)

H_1: "Alternative" hypothesis

Hypothesis generation with case series: This is a common way of forming hypothesis in clinical medicine. Case series involve the description of clinical/epidemiologic characteristics of a number of patients with a given disease. Usually a consecutive set of clinical cases of disease (or health issue) are taken and analyzed together to learn about the disease.

H_0: There is no association between the exposure and disease of interest

H_1: There is an association between the exposure and disease of interest (beyond what might be expected from random error alone)

Which study design helps forming a hypothesis? The answer is descriptive study designs as these provide enough of "raw material" that the researcher can use and frame a research question that can be tested via a hypothesis.

Correlational Hypothesis

This is a hypothesis that evolves after analyzing a dataset and correlations between variables can be planned.

Statistical test is clear (usually one per hypothesis) and the correlations are like this:

- X will positively relate to Y
- M will positively relate to Y
- X will positively relate to M
- X will not relate to Y when controlling for M

Bibliography

1. Formulate a research hypothesis. http:// study.com/academy/lesson/what-is-a-hypothesis-definition-lesson-quiz.html (Downloaded on 2nd May 2017).
2. Hypothesis and research question. http:// www.health.herts.ac.uk/immunology/ Web%20programme%20-%20Research health professionals/hypothesisresearch_question. htm (Downloaded on 2nd May 2017).
3. Research hypothesis. https://explorable.com/ research-hypothesis (Downloaded on 2nd May 2017).

Study Designs

Diseases do not come out of blue and the disease is not randomly distributed throughout a population. Hence a proper and systematic approach to study the differences in disease distribution in subgroups is needed. Study designs allow the study of causal and preventive factors. Basic question in analytic epidemiology is that if the expose and disease are linked or not. It is hence important to know what is exposure, who is exposed, what are potential health effects, what study design is needed to study the exposure and disease.

A clinical study design is a protocol of involving trials and experiments. However, most of the studies done by postgraduate students in medicine are observational studies so study designs cover them all. There are two major study designs: observational and experimental (Table 6.1).

Two major study designs have several types of subdesigns (Fig. 6.1).

Observations are easily made but are subject to bias and there could be systematic

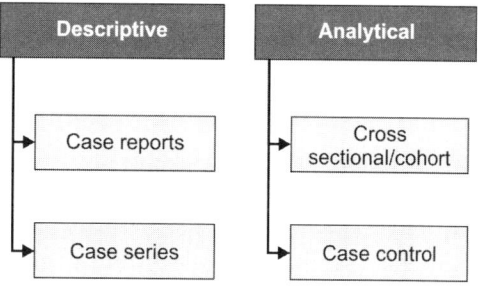

Fig. 6.1: Common study designs include case reports, which are the simplest ones to case series where some hypothesis can be generated as well. Case controls ad cross sectional studies can test the stated hypothesis in clinical medicine. However, in epidemiological studies, cohort studies are considered Gold Standards for testing hypothesis

error as well. However, some observations are less subject to bias than the others.

Experimental designs on the other hand are difficult to perform but are rewarding. These can provide definitive answers. Hence, the generalizability of experimental designs is more.

Table 6.1: Differences in observational and experimental designs

Observational	Experimental
• Non-experimental studies; observational because there is no intervention.	• Clinical trials are the most well known experimental design. Clinical trials use randomly assigned data; trials are planned study designs.
• Treatment and exposures occur in a "non-controlled" environment.	• Treatment and exposures occur in a "controlled" environment.
• Individuals can be observed prospectively, retrospectively, or currently	• Community trials use non-random data

Timelines of the Study

Prospective: Prospective studies are also called forward looking studies in which the researcher assembles a group of individuals who will be exposed to a risk factor or intervention and then waits to observe an outcome.

Retrospective: In retrospective (typically case control studies); the researcher elects a group of individuals expressly because they already experienced the outcome under study. It is then asked, in retrospect, if any of them have experienced certain events that they may have experienced certain events that may lead to the outcome.

Study Requirements

Before contemplating a study, one should be firmly establishing a study objective or hypothesis. Methods of assembling groups of study subjects, including developing specific case definition and avoiding systemic errors should be sorted before start of the study. One should be making valid and reliable observations, consideration of biased surveillance, blinding, and variability among observers. There should be some mechanism in place to deal with the same. Handling incomplete observations, such as individuals who are lost to follow-up, who fail to return questionnaire, or who appear to change their status during the study. Selecting appropriate comparison groups, including identifying and controlling for important factors that may impact on the study hypothesis and hence should be taken in account.

Ecology Study

This is a study based on group environment rather than individual environment. These studies are subject to ecologic fallacy. Ecologic variables may be used in many study designs, not just those that are cross sectional. They are frequently found in time series analyses.

Exploratory Studies

Exploratory studies are used when used when the state of knowledge about the phenomenon is poor. Generally, these are small scale studies, of limited duration. Their aim is to explore an unknown field. One could easily term such studies as "pilot" studies. Usually they are aimed to describe the phenomena hence are also called "descriptive studies".

Descriptive studies are usually done using surveys or questionnaires or scales and are often called 'statistical research'. The aim is to describe the data and characteristics about the population or phenomenon being studied. However, it does not answer questions how, when, and why the characteristics occurred. This has to be done using analytic research (e.g. case-control study).

Although the data description is factual, accurate and systematic, the research cannot describe what caused a situation or a phenomena, i.e. cause and effect relationship cannot be found. Thus, descriptive research cannot be used to create a causal relationship where one variable affects another. For example, using descriptive research one can say that employees who spend a lot of time in offices without sunlight are having low vitamin D_3 levels in their serum. However, if that itself is the cause can only be answered by case-control or cohort studies.

Analytic studies are used to test hypotheses at small or large scale. Examples include case-control; cohort and sometimes cross sectional studies can be used as analytic studies. Though a variety of study designs are used in biomedical and basic science but in medicine, the commonly used designs are given below (Table 6.2).

Case Reports

Case reports are the detailed presentation of a single case or handful of cases (generally two

Table 6.2: Common study designs

- Case reports
- Case series
- Cross sectional
- Case-control
- Cohort
- Randomized controlled clinical trial

or three). Generally, case reports describe a new or unique finding, e.g. previous undescribed disease, unexpected link between diseases, unexpected new therapeutic effect or, e.g. adverse events. These are often the starting point of someone getting started into medical writing.

Clinical Case-series

These are consecutive set of cases of a disorder/disease which derive from the practice of one or more healthcare professionals or healthcare setting. Clinical case series are of value in epidemiology for studying predictive symptoms, signs and tests. They are also useful for creating case definitions, clinical education, audit and research. They are hence very useful for health services research and establishing safety profiles (Table 6.3).

Table 6.3: Features of case series

- Group of patients with a similar diagnosis
- Assesses prevalent disease
- Cases may be identified from a single or multiple sources
- Report on new/unique condition
- Realistic design for rare disorders

Importance of Case Reports—Case Series in Medicine

Case reports and case series can be well received, and have significant influence on subsequent literature and possibly on clinical practice. Many are followed by clinical trials or by other epidemiological studies. Often, report rare conditions for which trials may not be feasible are reported as case reports or case series. One should however be wary of publication bias favouring positive results in case series. This may not always be the case though (Table 6.4).

Study Flow

Mostly an exploratory study can give us ideas about the variables that one can use to frame research question. Once a research question develops, then one can form a hypothesis

Table 6.4: Advantages and disadvantages of case series

Advantages

- Useful for hypothesis generation
- Informative for very rare disease with few established risk factors
- Characterizes averages for disorder

Disadvantages

- Cannot study cause and effect relationships
- Cannot assess disease frequency

and chose a study design depending upon hypothesis. The idea can be tested by cohort/case control or by clinical trials. Table 6.5 details the type of study designs and what they are supposed to do.

Table 6.5: Study designs and what they can explore

Descriptive	Case-control	Cohort	Clinical trials
Hypothesis developing study	Relation to outcomes can be investigated	Link with exposure can be studied	Proof of the found experimentally

Cross Sectional Study

Cross sectional study is a descriptive study in which disease and exposure status is measured simultaneously in a given population at a given time. Cross sectional studies can be thought of as providing a "snapshot" of the frequency and characteristics of a disease in a population at a particular point in time. This type of data can be used to assess the prevalence of acute or chronic conditions in a population. However, since exposure and disease status are measured at the same point in time, it may not be possible to distinguish whether the exposure preceded or followed the disease, and thus cause and effect relationships are not certain. It can measure prevalence and can show association between variables. However cause and effect cannot be determined.

Cross sectional study is often used to study conditions that are relatively frequent with long duration of expression (nonfatal, chronic conditions, e.g. diabetes, hypertension, etc.). Cross sectional study measures prevalence, not incidence of disease as there are no new cases. For example, community surveys done to know the prevalence of mental retardation in Delhi slums. It is not suitable for studying rare or highly fatal diseases or a disease with short duration of expression.

Though this is a common study design but the main disadvantages is that it is a weak observational study design. The temporal sequence of exposure and effect may be difficult or impossible to determine. In this type of study design, usually we do not know when disease occurred. If the event is rare then it is difficult to study. Quickly emerging diseases could be a problem as the incidence will count here rather than prevalence. Hence this study design is good for stable, chronic diseases with high prevalence.

Cohort Study

A cohort is a group of people who share a common characteristic or experience within a defined period. Thus a group of people who were born on a day or in a particular period, say 1974, form a birth cohort. The comparison group may be the general population from which the cohort is drawn, or it may be another cohort of persons thought to have had little or no exposure to the substance under investigation, but otherwise similar. Alternatively, subgroups within the cohort may be compared with each other.

Cohort study is also called longitudinal or prospective studies. So it is a forward looking study which aims to measure the incidence of the study. Cohort study starts with people free of disease and assesses exposure at "baseline" and then assesses disease status at "follow-up". This is in contrast to the case control study where the "case" is already present and the controls are chosen for the comparison. In cohort, there are no "cases" to begin with and it starts with healthy people.

Cohort study is a form of longitudinal observational study. It begins with a group of people who do not have the disease (share similar characters), takes baseline measurements,

then follows them overtime to determine whether uses correlations to determine the absolute risk of subject contraction.

Cohort is an example of an epidemiological question that can be answered by the use of a cohort study is does exposure to X (say, smoking) associate with outcome Y (say, lung cancer)? Such a study would recruit a group of smokers and a group of non-smokers (the unexposed group) and follow them for a set period of time and note differences in the incidence of lung cancer between the groups at the end of this time.

For example, in the group whose example is given above can be expanded as this: Doctors in the hospital treat patients with asthma and chronic obstructive lung disease but many of them do smoke also. Now we want to know the frequency of lung cancer in patients who smoke and who do not smoke if they are followed up for next 10 years. Of course, the frequency in the group which smokes will be much higher compared to the group that does not smoke. But still, some of the patients in the non smoker group may also develop lung cancer. Since these are going to be healthy individuals to start with and some of which may develop lung cancer; so we can calculate the incidence which cannot be calculated in the case-control/crosses sectional study as the disease has already occurred and we are tracking the patient to see what are possible risk factors.

Cohort studies are time consuming and are usually very expensive. However, they may have complete source population denominator and hence can calculate incidence rates or risks and their differences and ratios. Since a large number of subject are being followed for long; Cohort study design is convenient for studying many diseases.

When to do cohort study?

Cohort studies are good for determining cause and effect as they are longitudinal studies done overtime. Cohort study too can be nested with repeated measure design. When there is good evidence of exposure and disease (e.g. diabetes and dyslipidemia are associated).

It can be done when exposure is rare but incidence of disease is higher among exposed (bronchitis among pollution exposed). Additionally, this design is chosen when the follow-up is easy, as the cohort is stable or homogenous group. To start with, if we are contemplating cohort study, then both the cohorts (exposed/unexposed) are free of the disease. This is the major difference between case control studies and cohort where both groups are free from disease. That means, both the groups should equally susceptible to disease; the development of which can be studied in cohort. Both the groups should be comparable. Diagnostic and eligibility criteria for the disease should be defined well in advance. Components of cohort study are given in Table 6.6. Its strengths and weaknesses are given in Table 6.7.

Table 6.6: Components of cohort study

- Selection of study subjects
- Obtaining data on exposure
- Selection of comparison group
- Follow-up
- Analysis

Table 6.7: Strengths and weakness of cohort study

Strengths

- We can find out incidence rate and risk
- More than one disease related to single exposure
- Can establish cause-effect
- Good when exposure is rare
- Minimizes selection and information bias

Weaknesses of Cohort Study

- Loss to follow-up; attrition rates can be high
- Large sample needed
- Ineffective for rare diseases
- Expensive and time consuming.

Attributable Risk

Assume that we know a causal factor (e.g. diabetes for dementia) for a disease. Conceptually, the "attributable risk" for that factor is: difference in risk or incidence between exposed and unexposed people or the difference in risk or incidence between total population and unexposed people. For example, if diabetes is the vascular factor that can contribute to cognitive decline, then the risk produced by diabetes is attributable risk. Of course, this can be said only when we compared diabetic dementia patients with non-diabetic demented patients. We should have age matched controls too.

Attributable risk can be presented as: an "absolute" number, e.g. "80,000, or 20 per 100 cases/year of stroke are attributable to smoking" or a "relative" number, e.g. "20% of stroke cases are attributable to smoking".

Case-control Studies

Case-control studies are the types of observational studies in which two groups differing in outcomes are identified and compared on the basis of some supposed causal attributes or predictors. Case-control studies are often used to identify factors that may contribute to a medical condition by comparing subjects who have that condition/disease (cases) with patients who do not have the condition/disease (controls). Case-control studies are usually less expensive, and the sampling occurs from the source population. These studies can usually calculate only the ratio of incidence rates or risks. However, they are very useful for studying many exposures at the same time. It is important to know that case-control studies measure the exposure that has already happened and it is the exposure that is getting measured and compared among cases and controls. They have several characteristics:

- Observational/non-experimental
- Analytical
- Retrospective
- Proceed effect to cause
- Both exposure and disease have already occurred
- Uses comparison group.

Case control studies are good for diseases with long incubation period as one would not have to wait for long. This is in contrast to cohort where a longitudinal follow-up is needed and one would have to wait for long to know if the disease develops or not in those who are exposed. So, case-control studies can compress time and are fast to contemplate.

Clinically, case-control studies are usually done to elucidate the mechanism of disease. On a community level, they are done to measure the impact of exposure on the population. The decision to choose this design is taken knowing the characteristics of the exposure and disease, the current state of knowledge: The immediate goals of the study, research setting and the resources available are other predictors of the same. Control for extraneous variables is important and can be achieved by matching. Case-control study can be nested in a larger group called nested case-control study.

One of the best things while executing the case-control study is the economy, i.e. the study is not very expensive and is not time consuimg. Additionally, since many risk factors are under consideration, hence it is good for rare diseases. The results can only give approximations of actual rates with which the outcome occurs. The control group however should be carefully selected. Hypothesis development, establishment of definitions, case selections, control selection, and exposure determination are important steps in case-control studies. Its strengths and weaknesses are given in Table 6.8.

Disadvantages

1. Susceptible to bias if not carefully designed.

Table 6.8: Strengths and weaknesses of case-control study

Advantages
- Helps in uncovering etiology in rare diseases
- Important in understanding new diseases
- Commonly used in outbreaks investigation
- Useful if incubation period is long
- Relatively inexpensive

2. Especially susceptible to exposure misclassification.
3. Especially susceptible to recall bias.
4. Restricted to single outcome.
5. Incidence rates not usually calculate.
6. Cannot assess effects of matching variables.

Case Definitions

Case definition is critical in a case-control study. These definitions sould be operational. Patients with a specific outcome like presence of disease/hypertension needs to defined accurately so that it can be measured.

Controls

The controls should come from the population at risk of the disease. Naturally, men cannot be controls for a gynecological conditions and the controls should be "eligible for the exposure". That means, the controls should have same exposure rate as that of the population from where the cases are drawn. Table 6.9 details the types of controls.

Table 6.9: Types of controls
- Hospital or clinic control
- Dead control
- Controls with similar diseases
- Peer or case-nominated (friend/neighbour) control
- Population controls

Hospital controls
- Readily available hence commonly used
- Main reasons to use hospital controls are:
  - To select controls whose referral pattern is similar to cases
  - To obtain similar quality of examination
  - For convenience
- May not be representative of the population.

Principles of Selection of Controls

The study base should be such that the source of case and the control should be the same. Ideally, there should be similar misclassification errors in cases and controls. Also there should be same potential of recall bias in cases and control.

Association

Case control studies measure the associations and the strength of association can be measured in terms of odds ratio. Details have been given in the chapter on association. Following criteria should be fulfilled in case association were to be described.

- Criteria to be fulfilled:
  - Temporal association
  - Strength of association and effect of cessation
  - Specificity of association
  - Consistency of association
  - Biological plausibility
  - Coherence of association.

Clinical Trials

Clinical trials are experimental methods of testing hypotheses and not observational studies. In clinical trials, a concurrent, prospective comparison of two or more groups where one or more of the groups is deliberately exposed to an intervention, (usually drugs), while at least one group (the controls) is not exposed or receives a more standard therapy is done. The study groups are generated from a single, homogeneous pool of subjects (usually randomized). Assignment of individuals to each experimental or control group is determined by a method based on random events and without any consideration of which member of the pool is assigned to which group. It is important to know that all study participants (subjects, treating clinicians, and outcome evaluators) are unaware of which subjects are receiving an intervention and which are in a control group. This "blinding" may also extend to various participants being unaware of the true study hypothesis or the nature of the outcome measure. Control subjects receive an intervention that is either indistinguishable from the actual intervention or is felt to have equivalent impact in ways that might effect the outcome to be measured. This usually includes attention to psychological factors, such as the placebo or Hawthorne effects through which some outcomes of behavior may change because individuals believe that they are being treated or because they know that they are being observed. Remember, attention can affect performance. In general, control and experimental groups should both experience some form of intervention and have an equivalent amount of contact with the research staff.

Clinical trials are not done when multiple therapeutic modalities need to be investigated because too many subjects are needed to evaluate the many possible therapeutic combinations or there are small changes in a therapeutic plan (then effort it takes to do the study may outweigh the potential significances of the outcome). Therapies that are likely to become obsolete before the study is completed are not investigated in trials. Treatments with only rare outcomes or outcomes that will only be observable at a time far distant in the future.

QUASI-EXPERIMENTAL STUDIES

The inability to randomize individual study subjects could pose a problem in some studies. Additionally, there could be only a single study group available and no comparison group is there. If the pretesting is not available then one could do quasi-experimental studies. So basically these studies are studies with nonrandomized comparison group, where nonrandomized crossover is available.

Summary

The following is a very useful summary of research designs. It depends upon the nature of study, cost, time and the available resources. Of course the research should be ethically done.

Aim/objective	Types of studies
Observe/describe	• Descriptive, cross sectional • Case reports/case series • Surveys
Study predictors	• Case-control study • Cohort
Determine causes	• Twin studies

Cause and effect	• Double blind randomized trials
Explain	• Literature reviews
	• Systematic reviews
	• Meta-analysis
Testing tools	• Pilot study
Simple experimental designs	• Before and after studies
	• Randomized control trials
Complex experimental studies	• Factorial designs
	• Repeated measure designs

Bibliography

1. Chiao J. Culture–gene coevolution of individualism –collectivism and the serotonin transporter gene. *Proceedings of the Royal Society B 2009; 277,* 529–537. doi: 10.1098/rspb. 2009. 1650

2. Dunn EW, Aknin LB, Norton MI. Spending money on others promotes happiness. Science 2009; 319(5870), 1687–1688. doi:10. 1126/ science. 1150952

3. Festinger L, Riecken HW, Schachter S. (1956). When prophecy fails. Minneapolis, MN: University of Minnesota Press.

4. Harker LA, Keltner D. Expressions of positive emotion in women's college yearbook pictures and their relationship to personality and life outcomes across adulthood. Journal of Personality and Social Psychology, 2001; 80, 112–124.

5. King LA, Napa CK. What makes a life good? Journal of Personality and Social Psychology 1998; 75, 156–165.

6. Lucas RE, Clark AE, Georgellis Y, Diener E. Re-examining adaptation and the setpoint model of happiness: Reactions to changes in marital status. Journal of Personality and Social Psychology 2003; 84, 527–539.

7. Research designs. http://nobaproject.com/ modules/research-designs. (Accessed online dated 30th January 2017).

8. Research designs. https://explorable. com/ research-designs (Accessed online dated 30th January 2017).

9. Techniques of research designs. http://www. health.herts.ac.uk/immunology/Web% 20 programme%20-%20 Researchhealthprofessionals/ research_design.htm (Accessed online dated 30th January 2017).

Searching Literature

Learning objectives

Searching the literature is an art and science. This needs patience, practice and persistence. One has to take time to search as there are several related things that will come up in the sea of information. Searching relevant information can be challenging unless done methodically.

Literature Search

Searching medical literature methodically is important to answer a query. There are several web based and non-web tool available to help us do the same.

Why do Literature Search?

Healthcare includes the provision of information to professionals that is reliable, accurate, and up-to-date. Information explosion exists in the world today with billions of documents in the world wide web (www). Hence, it is hard to find the desired information at times but one would have to know which source is best for a specific situation.

Information search is more important nowadays, as there is an era of evidence-based practice, i.e. use medicines based on scientific evidence available. Systematic search strategy should be adopted when dealing with clinical questions to avoid 'information malpractice' as web contains all kind of information.

Why use web for Research?

Web is an extensive and an up-to-date resource. It not only offers convenience but it also has extra features, e.g. search facilities, links to other databases, supplementary information, etc. it has access to a wider range of material than might otherwise be available within the local medical library.

Web Library

Nowadays, web is the major source of information. Laptops, desktops, tablets, mobiles and I pads have become information collecting tools. Web library is any library or information resources that can be accessed electronically, e.g. electronic journals, databases, electronic books, hybrid digital collections, internet gateways and search engines or other free or fee-based medical access systems.

Electronic Journals

Both print and electronic versions of journals are in vogue nowadays. Electronic journals are web journals where full-text/whole journal is available online. These may have electronic version of print or electronic only journals (e-journals). Partial full-text/selected articles only could be published. At times they may have only table of contents/citations/abstracts or citations only. Electronic journals are of two main types (Table 7.1):

Table 7.1: Types of electronic journals

- Academic
  - Refereed journals
  - Review journals
  - Bulletins
- Non-academic
  - Magazines
  - Newspapers

Refereed Journals

Refereed journals disseminate research findings, and one could find out about research by others. It is easy to identify methodologies for own work by reading such journals (Table 7.2). This is because these are written by researchers and experts, that are aimed at researchers and experts. Also articles always cite sources and are peer reviewed; so one can read more about them as well.

Search Engine

Search engine is a program that searches documents for specified keywords and returns a list of documents where the keywords were found on the world wide web, a search engine utilizes automated robotics to gather and index information. Examples of the search engines include: Google (www.google.com) Google Scholar (www.scholar.google.com), pubmed (www.pubmed.com), etc. Each search engine offers something and it may have some shortcomings too (Table 7.3).

Table 7.2: Features of refereed journals

- Strengths/weaknesses
  - High-quality, reliable information
  - May be slow to be published due to review process
  - Often fee-based access/may be available via HINARI

Table 7.3: Advantages and disadvantages of common search engines

Google advantages	Google disadvantages
• Searches articles, books and webpages listen on goggle • Has advanced search options. • Can limit search by dates, document types, language, domain and more	No indexing terms • Huge retrieval of almost any topic • No ability to select citations for downloading or printing • Built in relevancy ranking based on times cited cannot limit to journal articles
Google scholar advantages	Google scholar disadvantages
• Searches journals, books and more academic sources • Can download individual citations into bibliographic managers • Contains citing information with links to sources citing a specific term	• No indexing terms • Huge retrieval of almost any topic • No ability to select citations for downloading or printing • Built in relevancy ranking based on times cited that • May result in bias toward older literature
Pubmed advantages	Pubmed disadvantages
• Well indexed using Medical Subject Headings (MeSH) • Can 'explode' terms • Contains 5,419 current journals in health sciences • Includes citations of e-journals prior to publication • Can download info to bibliographic managers • Can select citations to download or print	• Access limited almost exclusively to basic and health sciences journals that are indexed in the database • Does not search full-text of articles
CINAHL advantages	CINAHL disadvantages
• Well indexed and can 'explode' terms • Contains 2,960 journals in nursing and allied health plus books, dissertations and other items • Very current • Many ways of sorting retrieval • Can select citations to download or print	• Access limited to nursing and allied health materials that are indexed in the database • Does not search full-text for most items

Open Access Journals

'Open Access' (OA) journals are scholarly journals that are available without financial or technical barriers other than internet access. Articles either are directly accessible from the publisher (e.g. PLOS) or archived in a repository (e.g. PubMed Central). In most cases, the copyright is owned by the author, not the publisher. Some OA journals are subsidized by academic or governmental institutions.

Impact Factor

Impact factor of a journal is produced from Journal Citation Report (JCR), a product of Thomson Institute for Scientific Information (ISI). Impact factor is a measure reflecting the average number of citations to articles published in science and social science journals. It is calculated yearly for journals indexed in Thomson's *Journal Citation Reports.* It is used as a measure for the relative importance of a journal within its field; journals with higher impact factors are deemed to be more important than those with lower ones.

Searching the Literature

One should start with the keywords that describe the main idea of the topic/concept. Keywords are located in the *title, author, subject* or *abstract*, and journal fields, etc. One should use keyword searching when articles have not been indexed with subject headings. One may have to use synonyms (all the ways an author may have expressed and/or spelled the topic), e.g. back pain or back pains or backache or headache, etc.

Boolean Search

This is a search strategy that connect terms and locate records containing matching terms. Search terms are inserted in a search box– AND, OR, NOT. **Search terms** must be typed in UPPERCASE when used. Terms such as AND, NOT operators are processed in a left-to right sequence. These are processed first before the OR operators. OR operators are also processed from left-to-right. AND operator aims to combine two concepts and narrow a search. The **AND** operator is used to combine three concepts also, e.g. hip **AND** fracture **AND** elderly.

LEADING DATABASES/SEARCH DATABASES IN MEDICINES

1. Medline

Medline was developed by United States National Library of Medicine and has developed 16 different data bases that contain 12 million citations and author abstracts from over 4800 biomedical journals published in US and 70 other countries. This number keeps growing.

This is also called Medical Literature Analysis and Retrieval System or MEDLARS. One of these data bases is called MEDLINE. It is a bibliographic file of articles, and it is the most comprehensive, economical and widely used system in the world. Citations in MEDLINE are assigned subject headings from the MeSH vocabulary to assist users in their searches.

2. Pubmed (www.pubmed.com)

PubMed, a service of the National Library of Medicine (NLM), provides access to over 11 million citations from MEDLINE (the NLM's premier bibliographic database covering the fields of medicine, nursing, dentistry, veterinary medicine, the healthcare system, and preclinical sciences) and additional life sciences journals. PubMed includes links to many sites providing full text articles and other related sources. PubMed provides access to bibliographic information that includes MEDLINE, OLDMEDLINE, as well as: the out-of-scope citations (e.g. articles on plate tectonics or astrophysics) from certain MEDLINE journals, primarily general science and chemistry journals, for which the life sciences articles are indexed for MEDLINE.

3. Cochrane Reviews

The Cochrane Collaboration is an international non-profit and independent organization, dedicated to making up-to-date, accurate information about the effects of healthcare readily available worldwide. It produces and disseminates systematic reviews of health-care interventions and promotes the search for evidence in the form of clinical trials and other studies of interventions. The Cochrane Collaboration was founded more than 20 years back and named for the British epidemiologist, Archie Cochrane. The major product of the Collaboration is the Cochrane Database of Systematic Reviews which is published quarterly as part of The **Cochrane Library.** Those who prepare the reviews are mostly healthcare professionals who volunteer to work in one of the many **Collaborative Review Groups,** with editorial teams overseeing the preparation and maintenance of the reviews, as well as application of the rigorous quality standards for which Cochrane Reviews have become known. One should be wary of publication bias though.

Bibliography

1. Dupras DM, Ebbert JO. Clinicians' guide to new tools and features of PubMed. Mayo Clin Proc. 2007 Apr;82(4):480–483; quiz 484.

2. Ebbert JO, Dupras DM, Erwin PJ. Searching the medical literature using PubMed: a tutorial. Mayo Clin Proc. 2003 Jan;78(1):87–91.

3. Sood A, Erwin PJ, Ebbert JO. Using advanced search tools on PubMed for citation retrieval. Mayo Clin Proc. 2004 Oct;79(10):1295–1299; quiz 1300.

Chapter 8

Subject Selection

Learning objectives

A chosen sample may be taken by one of the several methods described in the chapter. However, the bottom line is the representativeness. If a sample is not representative, then the purpose gets defeated. Simple random is the simplest way in which it can be achieved. Several others are used too in given situations. The trick lies in hypothesis, study design, feasibility, duration, etc.

Sample Selection

A sample is "a smaller but representative collection of units from a population used to determine truths about that population" (Field, 2005). There are various steps needed in sampling of the study subjects.

Why Take a Sample?

Taking a sample and doing research is cheaper as it can be done at a lower cost. Additionally, one can ensure greater accuracy of results if the sample is representative. Speed of data collection could be fast. Again if the sample is selected well then one can ensure that almost all elements of the population have been included. However in some situations like counting of population, a census has to be done.

One has to start with definition of target population followed by the selection of a sampling frame (*see* below). After that one should decide what kind of sampling is needed; probability or nonprobability sampling. The sampling unit should be clear as it is a non-divisible unit (*see* below). The errors should be looked into and these could be related to both samples (random sampling error/chance fluctuations) or could be non sampling (e.g. faults in study designs).

Why Sample?

Resources like time, and money needed for research could be scarce and the workload could be substantial. A sample gives results with known accuracy that can be calculated mathematically.

Target Population

The population to be studied/to which the investigator wants to generalize his results, e.g. diabetics in Delhi or malnutrition in slum area.

Sampling Unit

Smallest unit is the unit from which sample can be selected. A **sampling unit** is one of the **units** into which an aggregate is divided for the purpose of **sampling**, each **unit** being regarded as individual and indivisible when the selection is made. For example, while studying stress among medical students; a single medical student could be a sampling unit.

Sampling Frame

List of all the sampling units from which sample is drawn.

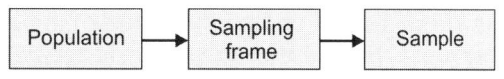

Sampling Scheme

This is the method of selecting sampling units from sampling frame. It starts by asking what is the population? What are the parameters of interest? What is the sampling frame? What is the type of sample and what size sample is needed? Lastly, how much will it cost?

SAMPLING METHODS

Sampling Population

It is important to as to what is population of interest? To whom do you want to generalize the results? Population of interest could be all doctors, school children, Indians as a whole, women aged 15–45 years and lot of others. However, one cannot study the population as a whole. One would have to take a fraction of the whole population. Sampling procedure and participation (response) could affect the sample to be taken for study. When population is very small, and when does not expect a very high response; then population as a whole could be taken as well. Census is also another example where whole population has to be taken. Two major types of sampling are given below (Table 8.1).

Table 8.1: Major types of sampling procedures

Probability	Non-probability
• Systematic	• Convenience
• Simple random	• Snow ball-Judgement
• Cluster	• Quota

Sampling could be of many types: broadly, it is of two main types: probability and non-probability sampling.

Probability Sampling

Probability sampling is a sampling technique in which every member of the population will have a known, nonzero probability of being selected. This form of selection utilizes random selection. The tool of selecting individuals by this method should be such that there are equal probability of being chosen, e.g. flipping through a coin, lottery, etc.

Non-probability Sampling

Non-probability sampling employs no statistical techniques for measuring random sampling error in a non-probability sample. Therefore,

generalizability is **never** statistically appropriate. Units of the sample are chosen on the basis of personal judgment or convenience. The selection is based upon the subjective judgment of the researcher rather than selection methods.

Simple Random Sampling

Sample random sampling assures that each element in the population has an equal chance of getting selected. Random number generator could be used. This sample is considered to be unbiased and supposed to have independence. Each individual has an equal chance of getting selected.

Probability of selection is = sample size/ population size

Advantages of simple random method is that minimal knowledge of population needed. Both external and internal validity are high.

The disadvantage is high cost; low frequency of use and needs a sampling frame. It does not use researchers' expertise. However, it may have a larger risk of random error than stratified random sampling.

The selection of subjects can be done by picking up a random number and the select the rest of the subjects in a random fashion. Figure 8.1 gives the details in a diagrammatic manner. Likewise, the same can be done using table of random number which can

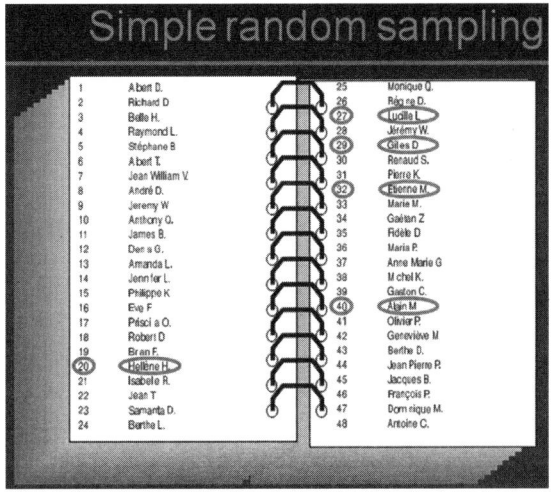

Table of random numbers

6 8 4 2 5 7 9 5 4 1 2 5 6 3 2 1 4 0

5 8 2 0 3 2 1 5 4 7 8 5 9 6 2 0 2 4

3 6 2 3 3 3 2 5 4 7 8 9 1 2 0 3 2 5

9 8 5 2 6 3 0 1 7 4 2 4 5 0 3 6 8 6

be generated easily using MS Excel or www.randomization.com.

Systematic Random Sampling

This is a type of probability sampling in which every kth member of the population is selected (sampling interval). The principle of selection is same as that of the simple random as the *p-value* and confidence interval are calculated same way (Fig. 8.1).

$$\text{Sampling fraction} = \frac{\text{Actual sample size}}{\text{Total population}}$$

Sampling interval = k = N/n
N = size of the population
n = sample size

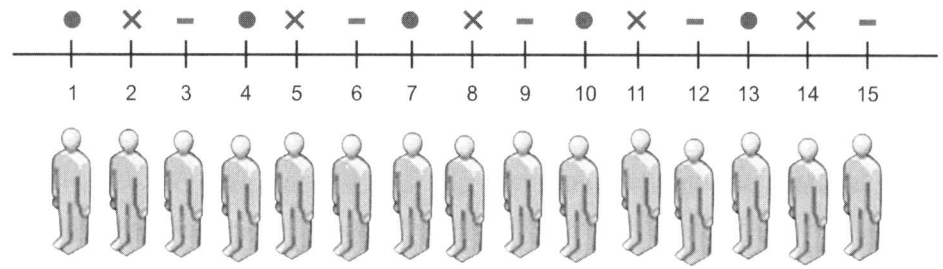

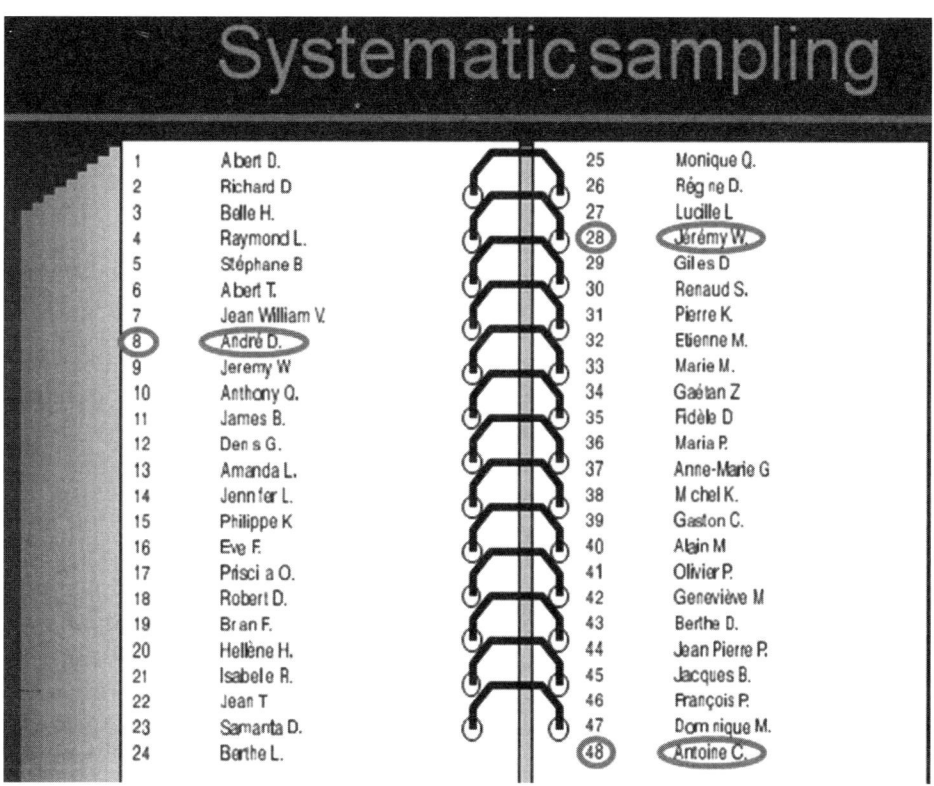

Fig. 8.1: A common example of systematic example

For example, if we want to obtain a sample of 100 from a population of 1,000. One would have to select every, 10th (or kth) person from the list.

$$k = 1000/100 = 10$$

Systematic random sampling is random sampling done systematically. The initial starting point is selected by a random process, and then every nth number on the list is selected. Sampling interval or n is selected. The number of population elements between the units selected for the sample.

Advantages of systematic random include moderate cost; moderate usage and the external and internal validity is high; statistical estimation of error is possible. The sample is simple to draw sample and is easy to verify. The disadvantages include periodic ordering and requires a large sampling frame. Another problem is that complete list of units must be available in order to select them systematically.

Stratified Random Sampling

This is a method of sampling that involves division of the study population into smaller groups which are called strata. These are formed based upon attributes or characters, e.g. age wise division, income wise, education wise, etc. These are then pooled to form a random sample which can be chosen for the study.

Stratified random sampling is of two types:

1. *Proportional stratified sample*: The number of sampling units drawn from each stratum is in proportion to the relative population size of that stratum. For example, if the group represents 15% of the population, the stratum representing that group will comprise 15% of the sample.

2. *Disproportional stratified sample*: The number of sampling units drawn from each stratum is allocated according to analytical considerations, e.g. as variability increases sample size of stratum should increase.

Advantages of stratified random sampling include representation of all groups in sample population needed. Characteristics of each stratum can be estimated and comparisons could be made. This method reduces variability as different strata have been pooled. Disadvantages include need of accurate information on proportions of each stratum and stratification could be costly and time consuming.

Cluster Sampling

Cluster sampling is a sampling technique when we have to study naturally available heterogeneous groups. It is used in community and marketing research. The whole population is divided in clusters and a simple random sample is selected.

Clusters are easier to obtain than a simple random or systematic sample of the same size.

In cluster sampling, the primary sampling unit is not the individual element, but a large cluster of elements (e.g. slums/houses). Either the cluster is randomly selected or the elements within are randomly selected.

It can be area sampling or multistage sampling. Area sample include primary sampling unit as is a geographical area. Multistage area sample involves a combination of two or more types of probability sampling techniques. Typically, progressively smaller geographical areas are randomly selected in a series of steps.

Advantages include low cost and high yield of data. However, it requires list of all clusters, but only of individuals within chosen clusters. Importantly, it can estimate characteristics of both cluster and population. Disadvantages include larger error for comparable size than other probability methods. Multistage could be very expensive and validity depends on other methods used. Additionally, clusters lead to violation that the subjects are independent units. Homogeneity and heterogeneity has to be kept in mind. Figures 8.2 to 8.4 explain this process diagrammatically.

Type 1 Error

The probability of finding a difference with our sample compared to population, and there really is not one. This is also known as the á

Cluster sampling

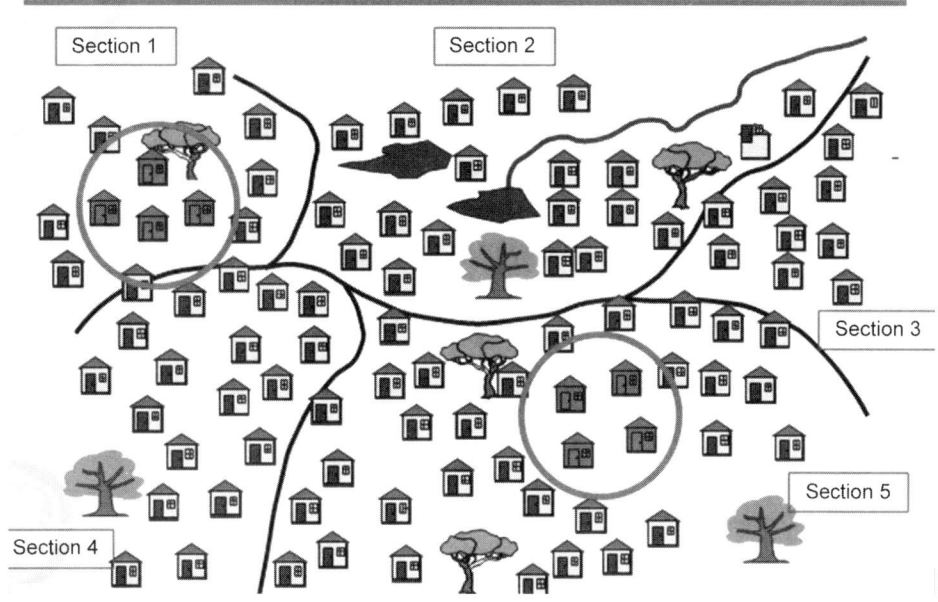

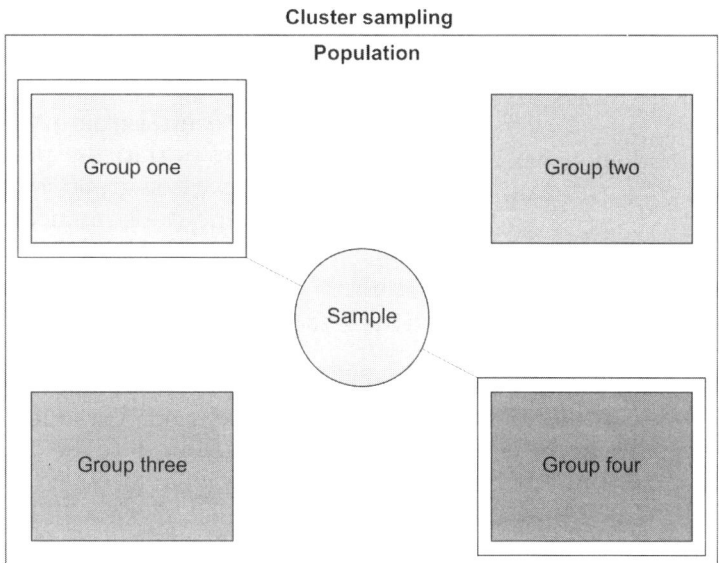

Fig. 8.2: An example of forming clusters

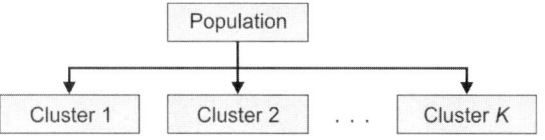

Fig. 8.3: Selecting clusters

(or "type 1 error"). This is the probability of committing an error that may have serious consequences for drug research. Usually it is set at 5% (or 0.05).

Type 2 Error

The probability of not finding a difference that actually exists between our sample compared to the population. This is known as the β (or "type 2 error"). This occurs when we miss the difference or are unable to spot the difference. Power is $(1-\beta)$ and is usually 80%.

Sampling Error

Sampling error is the degree to which a given sample differs from the underlying population. Sampling error tends to be high with small sample sizes and will decrease as sample size increases. So, the simplest way to reduce sampling error is to increase sample size. To be able to reduce the sampling error, the group to which you wish to generalize the results of the study should be defined as specifically as possible.
- Systematic error (or bias)
  - Inaccurate response (information bias)
  - Selection bias
- Sampling error (random error).

Sample Size

The size of the sample for a study should be large enough to show clinically relevant differences between study groups with statistical significance, and small enough to be practical and feasible. Using confidence intervals (as opposed to *p-value* only) allows the investigator not only to reject or accept a hypothesis within a known degree of uncertainty, but also to estimate the size of the treatment effect together with some measure of the uncertainty in the estimate. Attrition of subjects should be considered in advance.

Loss to Follow-up

Attrition rates greater than 30% make interpretation of the results very difficult. The original estimates of adequate sample size must take into account.

Convenience Sampling

Convenience sampling is ease of access and the sample is selected from elements of a population that are easily accessible. Snowball sampling means the friend of friend is selected. Purposive sampling is also called judgemental sampling where one chooses who you think should be in the study. In the quota sampling, the probability of being chosen is unknown. This is however cheaper- but unable to generalise. Therefore, there is a potential for bias.

Assigning Groups

  a. Case control group: A proper comparison requires that the performance of the comparison group is an adequate proxy for the performance of the treatment group if they had not received the intervention.

  b. Random allocation; the groups are same with respect to the dependent variable before the independent variable was introduced. Variables other than those considered to be independent and dependent through the life of study.

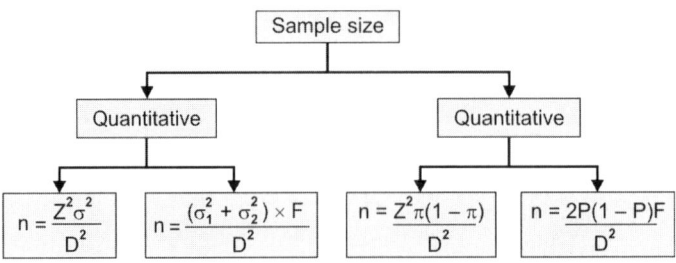

Fig. 8.4: Common formulae for sample sizes

Matching

a. *Pair matching*: It is a specific match, in which comparison subject is found for each intervention subject.

b. *Non-paired matching*: There is no attempt is made to find specific comparison subjects for each intervention subjects.

c. *Frequency matching*: The distribution of the confounding variable in the experimental intervention group is stratified, and one attempts to equalize the number of experimental intervention and comparison subjects in each stratum.

d. *Mean matching*: Attempts are made to match the sample means for the confounding variable in question.

Problem 1

A study is to be performed to determine a certain parameter in a community. From a previous study a SD of 46 was obtained.

If a sample error of up to 4 is to be accepted. How many subjects should be included in this study at 99% level of confidence?

Answer

$$n = \frac{Z^2 \sigma^2}{D^2}$$

$$n = \frac{2.58^2 \times 46^2}{4^2} = 880.3 \sim 881$$

Problem 2

- A study is to be done to determine effect of 2 drugs (A and B) on blood glucose level. From previous studies using those drugs, SD of BGL of 8 and 12 g/dl were obtained respectively.

- A significant level of 95% and a power of 90% is required to detect a mean difference between the two groups of 3 g/dl. How many subjects should be include in each group?

Answer

$$n = \frac{\left(\sigma_1^2 + \sigma_2^2\right) \times F}{D^2}$$

$$n = \frac{\left(8^2 + 12^2\right) \times 10.5}{3^2} = 242.6 \sim 243$$

in each group

Problem 3

It was desired to estimate proportion of anemic children in a certain preparatory school. In a similar study at another school a proportion of 30 % was detected.

Compute the minimal sample size required at a confidence limit of 95% and accepting a difference of up to 4% of the true population.

Answer

$$n = \frac{Z^2 \pi (1 - \pi)}{D^2}$$

$$n = \frac{1.96^2 \times 0.3 (1 - 0.3)}{(0.04)^2} = 504.21 \sim 505$$

Problem 4

In previous studies, percentage of hypertensives among diabetics was 70% and among non-diabetics was 40% in a certain community.

A researcher wants to perform a comparative study for hypertension among diabetics and non-diabetics at a confidence limit 95% and power 80%, what is the minimal sample to be taken from each group with 4% accepted difference of true value?

Answer

$$n = \frac{2P(1 - P)F}{D^2}$$

$$n = \frac{2 \times 0.55(1 - 0.55) \times 7.8}{0.04^2} = 2413.2$$

Bibliography

1. Karthik S, Sanjeev V. Thomas, Geetha S. Design, data analysis and sampling techniques for clinical research. Ann Indian Acad Neurol. 2011 Oct-Dec; 14(4): 287–290. doi: 10.4103/0972-2327.91951

2. Ranstam J. Sampling uncertainty in medical research. http://www.sciencedirect.com/science/article/pii/S1063458409001071.

3. Sampling in Medical Research. *Br Med J* 1953; 2 doi: https://doi.org/10.1136/bmj.2.4849.1284 (Published 12 December 1953).

Causality in Medical Research

Learning objectives

Causality is nothing but a relationship among the variables under study. However, it should not be interpreted that causal relationship means that change in one variable should automatically lead to the change in the other variable too. This is because the variables are inter-related. Causation indicates that one event in question occurs as a result of occurrence of the other, i.e. A causes B. This implies that there is a causal relationship between variables. Almost all of statistics is an attempt to discover whether two variables are associated, and if so, how strongly, and whether chance can explain the observed association. Statistics are primarily designed to assess the role of chance in that association. A *p-value* only tells us how unlikely the association is to have arisen by chance.

INTRODUCTION

Causality is a concrete sequence of causally linked events. As per a dictionary meaning of the word; causality is a relationship between variables where A precedes and causes B. This is enhanced if an exposure is associated with a specific disease, and not with whole variety of diseases.

Causality is also enhanced if a disease is associated with a specific exposure, and not with a whole variety of exposures. Though causality is most sought after thing in medicine where we tend to look for cause and effect; there are several drawbacks of the same. For example, the causation may be limited, subject to modification, sometimes not measureable and may even be subjective at times! The "criteria" may be really guidelines and not be binding.

Association

This is a relationship between two variables, whether dependent or not. It is important to know that merely the presence of association need not to be causal.

Associations can be real or spurious. Association is likely to be causal if the cause is distributed at same level as the factors and the incidence is much higher in the exposed population. Exposure is more frequent than the disease should follow exposure. Also the causality is likely when it is dose dependent, expected response, and other cause-effect should be ruled out before labeling A as the cause of B. Additionally, a proof of causality comes when controlling A should result in decreased incidence of B.

Mere presence of association is less meaningful compared to the implication of it, i.e. the association of the factor should fit the biological knowledge as well. One must look for support in the laboratory, or from other aspects of the biology of the condition. Causes, such as molecular cause, physiological cause, personal cause and social cause should be looked into. In essence in medicine, the "cause" from the perspective of several or aspects of the environment, broadly defined, if removed or controlled, would reduce the burden of disease. This is the major aim of determining the causality.

DETERMINISTIC CAUSALITY

Many scientists expect a cause to be very closely related to an effect, as in necessary and sufficient causes:

Necessary cause: The cause must be present for the outcome to happen. However, the cause can be present without the outcome happening, e.g. sun exposure and sun-burns.

Sufficient cause: If the cause is present the outcome must occur. However, the outcome can occur without the cause being present, e.g. includes low sun exposure and low vitamin D status.

Necessary

If outcomes are defining in terms of causes, the cause is necessary by definition. For example, the tubercle bacillus is necessary for tuberculosis by the definition of tuberculosis. Etiologic (as contrasted to manifestation) classification of diseases often produces necessary causes.

Hepatitis B once looked to be a necessary cause of hepatocellular carcinoma. But now we see that hepatitis C may produce it too.

Sufficient

Sufficient causes are very rare in medicine, because it is exceptional that one exposure is by itself enough to cause disease. Usually exposures are much more common than the diseases they cause. Only about 5% of people who smoke get lung cancer. Likewise, only a handful of people who are exposed to air pollution will get asthmatic attacks. The measles virus virtually always causes people to get clinical measles, and rabies infection is always fatal.

HIV could once be classified as both the necessary and sufficient cause of AIDS. Now, however, it may be that one can be infected with HIV and never get AIDS, either because of rare genetic protection, or because of treatment of the virus. Koch's postulates were an example of deterministic causality. To prove that an organism causes a disease, he required that:

1. The organism must be isolated in every case of the disease (i.e. be necessary).

2. The organism must be grown in pure culture.

3. The organism must always cause the disease when inoculated into an experimental animal (i.e. be sufficient).

4. The organism must then be recovered from the experimental animal and identified.

Probabilistic Causality

In epidemiology, most causes have much weaker relationships to effects. For example, high cholesterol may lead to heart disease, but it need not (insufficient), and heart disease does not require a high cholesterol (unnecessary). The emphasis on multiple causes in probabilistic causality leads to expressions, such as the web of causation, or chain of causation.

The measures of association-odds ratio, risk ratio, or correlation coefficient, and of public health impact, e.g. population attributable risk—are related to the strength of the causal relationship. The higher the odds ratio, the closer the cause is to being necessary and sufficient.

A population attributable risk of 100% means that the cause is necessary—all cases would be prevented if the cause were removed.

One pragmatic definition of a cause or determinant of a disease is an *exposure* which produces a regular and predictable change in the risk of the disease, e.g. smoking status and lung cancer.

Association vs Causation

To decide whether exposure A causes disease B, we must first find out whether the two variables are associated, i.e. whether one is found more commonly in the presence of the other. An example of such a relationship could be diabetes and hypertension.

It should be noted that the statistical analysis alone cannot constitute proof of a causal relationship. The process of weighing evidence at the level of the individual is clinical judgment (e.g. should this patient with a urinary tract infection be treated with one antibiotic or other?). The process of weighing evidence at the level of the population is epidemiological judgment (e.g. men over 45 should take aspirin daily to prevent heart attacks). When looking at data from epidemiological studies, we often use casual criteria to assist in weighing the evidence.

Checking Association

One should look at selection or measurement bias and if it is not present, then confounding should be ruled out. Then one can apply guidelines for casual associating and if the guidelines so indicates, a causal relationship can be found. Alternative explanation for the phenomena should not be present.

The following guidelines should be satisfied if the causality needs to be assessed:

Consistency: Is the same association found in many studies? Hundreds of studies have shown that smoking and lung cancer are associated, and no serious study has failed to show this association. But whether oral contraceptives are associated with breast cancer is uncertain because some studies show an association, but others do not. Meta-analysis is a formal method to assess the consistency of the measure of association across many studies.

Consistency can mean either be the exact replication, as in the laboratory sciences, or replication under many different circumstances. In epidemiology, exact replication is impossible. The repeated observation of an association in studies conducted on different populations under different circumstances. If the studies conducted by different researchers, at different times, in different settings on different populations using different study designs and if all produce consistent results, then this strengthens the argument for causation. Example includes the association between cigarette smoking and lung cancer that has been consistently demonstrated in a number of different types of epidemiological study (ecological, case-control, cohort).

Strength of Association

One of the important question in causation is that if the association strong was? Heavy smoking is associated with a twenty-fold higher rate of lung cancer, and a doubled rate of heart disease. The association of smoking with lung cancer is therefore stronger than its association with heart disease. The stronger the association the more likely it is to be truly causal. One reason for the importance is that any confounding variable must have a larger association with the outcome to be confounding. The larger the relative risk observed, the less likely it is that a confounder with an even larger relative risk is lurking in the background.

Measures of Association

This is used to quantify the strength of the association between an exposure and outcome, e.g. relative risk, odds ratio. Strong associations are more likely to be causal than weak associations. The larger the Relative Risk (RR) or Odds Ratio (OR), the greater the likelihood that the relationship is causal. Weak associations are more likely to be explained by undetected biases or confounders.

Temporality

Temporality refers to the necessity for the exposure to precede the outcome (effect) in time. Any claim of causation must involve the cause preceding in time the presumed effect. This is easier to establish in certain study designs, e.g. prospective cohort study. It is important to know that the lack of temporality rules out causality.

Dose Response Curve

Dose response is also called the biological gradient. This just means that "higher the dose, greater is the chance of likelihood". In quantitative terms, the relationship between the amount of exposure (dose) to a substance and the resulting changes in outcome (response).

If a regular gradient of disease risk is found to parallel a gradient in exposure (e.g. light smokers get lung cancer at a rate intermediate between non-smokers and heavy smokers) the likelihood of a causal relationship is enhanced. Dose-response is generally thought of as a sub-category of strength.

However, dose-response is not relevant to all exposure-disease relationships, because disease sometimes only occurs above a fixed threshold of exposure, and thus a dose-response relationship need not be seen. (remember also that misclassification of adjacent classes can easily produce an apparent dose-response relationship).

Biological Plausibility

Biological plausibility refers to the biological plausibility of the hypothesised causal relationship between the exposure and the outcome. A relationship is biological plausible if it asks if there is a logical and plausible biological mechanism to explain the relationship?

Checking Causality

a. **Strength of association:** "The lung cancer rate for smokers was quite a bit higher than for non-smokers (e.g. one study estimated that smokers are about 35% more likely than non-smokers to get lung cancer)".

b. **Temporality:** Smoking in the vast majority of cases preceded the onset of lung cancer.

c. **Consistency:** Different methods (e.g. prospective and retrospective studies) produced the same result. The relationship also appeared for different kinds of people (e.g. males and females).

d. **Theoretical plausibility:** Biological theory of smoking causing tissue damage which overtime results in cancer in the cells was a highly plausible explanation.

e. **Dose response relationship:** Data showed a positive, linear relationship between the amount smoked and the incidence of lung cancer.

f. **Experimental evidence:** Tar painted on laboratory rabbits' ears was shown to produce cancer in the ear tissue overtime. Hence, it was clear that carcinogens were present in tobacco tar.

g. **Analogy:** Induced smoking with laboratory rats showed a causal relationship. It, therefore, was not a great jump for scientists to apply this to humans.

Bibliography

1. Bradford-Hill A. The environment and disease: Association or causation? *Proc R Soc Med.* 1965; 58:295–300.
2. Doll R. Sir Austin Bradford Hill and the progress of medical science. British Medical Journal. 1991; 305:1521–1526.
3. Grimes DA. Cause and effect - or coincidence? *Contemporary OB/GYN Jan* 1984:109–115.
4. Hill AB. The environment and disease: Association or causation. Proceedings of the Royal Society of Medicine 1965; 58:295–300.
5. Hill BA. The environment and disease: Association or causation? Proceedings of the Royal Society of Medicine. 1965; 58:295–300.
6. Paneth N. Causal inference. Michigan State University.
7. Peterson HB, Kleinbaum DG. Interpreting the literature in Obstetrics and Gynecology: I. Key concepts in epidemiology and biostatistics. *Obstet Gynecol.* 1991; 78(4):710–717.
8. Porta M. A dictionary of epidemiology. New York, Oxford: Oxford University Press, 2008.
9. Rizzi DA, Pedersen SA. Causality in medicine: towards a theory and terminology. *Theor Med.* 1992 Sep; 13(3):233–254.
10. Rothman J, Greenland S. Modern epidemiology. Second edition. Lippincott-Raven Publishers, 1998.
11. Rothman KJ (editor). Causal inference. Chestnut Hill: Epidemiology Resources Inc., 1988.
12. Susser M. Judgement and causal inference: Criteria in epidemiologic studies. American Journal of Epidemiology. 1977; 105:1–15.
13. Susser MW. What is a cause and how do we know one? A grammar for pragmatic epidemiology. American Journal of Epidemiology 1991; 133: 635–648.

Protocol Writing

Learning objectives

A protocol is the first document that a student deals within clinical/medical research. This is very important piece of work and has to be meticulously worked. This is detailed set of activity that one would propose and these are supported by evidence and preliminary evidence. It is a practical schedule of timetable that should show title, aim, objectives, material methods and what are actually trying to achieve.

A protocol is a document that describes the objective/s, design, methodology, statistical considerations, and organisation of the trial. Usually, the protocol also gives the background and rational for the trial (Table 10.1). National Institute of Health, USA defines protocol as a "complete written description of, and scientific rationale for, a research activity involving human subjects". The structure of the protocol is given in Table 10.2.

General considerations

In general the protocol should be candid about the procedure, i.e. the protocol should clearly state that the trial involves research. The purpose of the research or trial and its experimental aspects should be made clear. If it is clinical trial; then the treatments and probability for random assignment to each treatment should explicitly be stated. Trial procedures to be followed and Subject's responsibilities have to be delineated. Importantly, the risks, inconveniences, and benefits to the subject have to be clearly stated, also the alternative treatments available from which the subjects can choose should be made available. It is imperative that the participation in the research has to be done out of the free will and the subjects should not be unduly influenced to participate. They should be fully informed of all pertinent aspects of the study. Written information should be as non-technical as possible so that it can be understood well. Subjects must be given ample time to ask questions. The consent to participate should be signed and personally dated by the subject (or his/her legally acceptable representative) and by the person who conducted the informed consent discussion.

Structure

A protocol should be structurally well planned. Any haphazardness can put off the evaluators. If this is a project protocol to be submitted to the funding agency, it should be very meticulous (Tables 10.1 and 10.2).

Table 10.1: Components of protocol

- Objectives
- Design
- Methodology

Table 10.2: Structure of research protocol

- Introduction/abstract
- Objectives (including study schema)
- Background/rationale
- Eligibility criteria
- Study design/methods (including drug/device info)
- Safety/adverse events
- Regulatory guidance
- Statistical section (including analysis and monitoring)
- Human subjects protection/informed consent

Need for Protocol

We need a protocol for a number of reasons, e.g. scientific validity, subject safety provisions and replicate the science behind the research if necessary. Also it is needed for regulatory requirements. Without a protocol, a research is headless. For master's and doctoral students, protocol is not only serves as a starting point for beginning the study but it will be needed at the time of submission of thesis too.

Writing Protocol

This is a matter of judgement and the gross rule of thumb is to include the right amount of detail necessary for the reader of each section to be able to understand exactly what is required to conduct the study.

Who can Write Protocol?

Protocols can be written by students, sponsors, and investigators. All protocols however, will differ from each other.

- *Sponsor*
  - Commercial manufacturer
    - Pharmaceutical or biotech company.
    - Medical device company.
- *Investigators and study team*
  - Investigator initiated (e.g. a doctor seeing bronchitis patients wants to study the frequency of such episodes during Delhi winters).
  - Investigator in collaboration with investigators at another institution.

Industries sponsored protocols
- Protocol generally part of larger investigational plan to get the drug/device approved by approval agency (Food and Drug Administration).
  - Large multi-centric trials
  - Protocol is complex
  - Study design is decided by sponsor
- *Centralized research activities*
  - Data analysis
  - FDA reporting
  - May use a central lab

- *Funding*
  - Sponsor pays for research activities
  - Contract between sponsor, institute and investigator (tripartite).

Investigator Initiated Research (IAR)

Investigators plan research and may have independently conceived and developed ideas. These ideas developed by scientists become the parts of research projects. They may range from a small pilot study to large multi-site clinical trials. Such projects may study a disease process or an intervention. It is important to know that the investigator are responsible for all research activities including, reporting to funding and oversight entities, data analysis and of course the publications of the report. Funding of the research can be done by the various companies, e.g. pharmaceutical, biotech, medical device, etc.

Protocol Types

There are three general types of protocols, e.g. retrospective review—where the review of the existing literature is done (usually with data). Second type is natural history study—may get tissues and DNA samples, etc. The third type is interventional—where the phase I/II, phase III, phase IV studies are done. As a principal investigator, one would have to figure out if the project was reasonable and if the resources were available or not. The risks to the population will have to be sorted as well.

One may have to include an associate investigator who could be important in conducting the research.

Audience

One would have to keep the "audience" in mind (the group who will evaluate the protocol). These could be other physicians, nurses, clinical research associate; Institute Review Board (IRB) members, etc. there could be scientific reviewers too in this protocol review committee (Table 10.3).

Table 10.3: Protocol review committee

- IRB members
- Scientific reviewers

Protocol Templates

Many templates are available nowadays at the websites of professional institutes and bodies. Such programs encourage or require the use of protocol templates. Following the template guidelines can help guide authors, but not every part of a template will necessarily apply in a given study.

Objectives of Writing a Protocol

Objectives of writing a protocol should be stated clearly as hypotheses to be tested. Each objective should have a corresponding discussion in the statistical section.

Rationale of Writing a Protocol

All protocols require a section detailing the scientific rationale for a protocol and the justification in medical and scientific literature for the hypothesis being proposed. Introductory section should be as succinct as possible and should be organized in a logical, sequential flow.

Citations

One should double check all citations before finalizing. It should be noted that bibliographic inaccuracies harm the citing author and may cast doubt on the quality of the protocol or the research being reported. As a general rule it has been said that the authors should verify references against the original document. Being casual about the references can spoil the whole document.

Eligibility Criteria

Eligibility criteria are the largest barrier to accrual to clinical trials. Poorly written or poorly conceived criteria may undermine a trial's generalizability and scientific validity of the study. Eligibility criteria stated as either exclusion or inclusion criteria—define and limit the kinds of patients that can participate in a clinical trial. Reasons for imposing eligibility criteria can include scientific rationales, safety concerns, regulatory issues, and practical considerations. The criteria should not be too inclusive as there are problems with restrictive criteria such as limitations of generalizability, failure to mimic actual clinical practice, increased study complexity, increased costs, decreased patient accrual, etc.

Recommendations for constructing an acceptable criteria is that the number of eligibility criteria should be kept to a minimum. Also, the criteria should include only those absolutely necessary to ensure scientific validity and patient safety. Eligibility criteria should be clearly defined and verifiable by an external auditor. The criteria should be straightforward and unambiguous. Some groups are deliberately excluded from the protocols (Table 10.4).

Table 10.4: Groups excluded from clinical trials

- Pregnant and/or nursing women
- All women of childbearing age
- Elderly

A note can be given to make it a point that "Pregnant and/or nursing women are not eligible for this study. Also, all women of childbearing potential must have a negative pregnancy test (urine) within 2 weeks of study enrollment". While framing the eligibility criteria; one should be aware of the consequences of highly specific criteria. This can make enrollment difficult.

Study Design

The study design section of the protocol should contain a stepwise description of all procedures required by the study. A good study design section includes sufficient information for the participating site to develop a comprehensive clinical pathway for study patients. Parts of the study design section may include initial evaluations, screening tests, required lab tests, details of treatment and ancillary procedures, agent information or device specifications, dose scheduling and modification and calendars.

Safety Evaluation

The safety or adverse drug events section should include contain detailed information for reporting adverse events, including reporting to the FDA and/or the sponsor. The details should include blinding/unblinding processes (if applicable), lists of expected adverse events, etc. Human subject protection and provisions about ethical issues should be included.

This section on safety should includes the discussion of subject selection and exclusion, proposed methods of patient recruitment, recruitment (or exclusion) of special subjects, including vulnerable subjects, lists of potential risks and benefits, including justification for risks. All the information included should be up to date.

Case Record Form

Case record form is a document used to record data on which the reporting of the clinical trial/ study is done. It is very helpful for data analysis.

Purpose of the information collected in the case record form is to answer the hypothesis formulated in the study protocol and to provide relevant safety data relating to the study drug.

Case Record Form (CRF) should request the precise information required by the protocol. It should contain only the information required by the protocol. Also it should request the information in a way that completion is simple, relatively quick, and as unambiguous as possible, and that all assessment are straight forward to complete. Additionally, it should presents information as clearly as is possible to enable the investigator to review the subjects continuing eligibility.

Informed Consent

The office of human subjects research recognizes 3 fundamental conditions for a valid informed consent (Fig. 10.1):

a. Disclosure of relevant information to prospective research subjects.
b. Comprehension of the information provided.
c. Voluntary agreement of the subject, free from coercion.
d. Proxy consent if mentally ill.

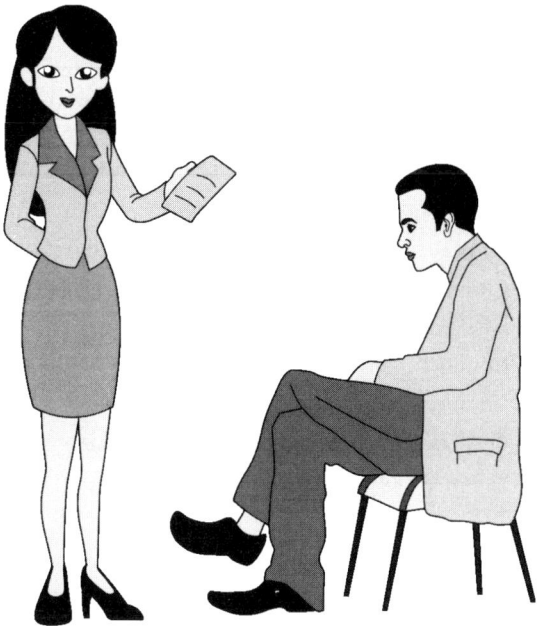

Fig. 10.1: Obtaining consent is a scientifically sound procedure and needs to be done following all guidelines

e. **Disclosure of relevant information:** All the information related to the research project, its procedure, reporting, inclusion and exclusion should be provided.

f. **Comprehension of the information provided:** Subjects should be informed of the risk, benefits and ay contingency if it arises should be informed as well. It should be provided in a language easily understood by the participants.

g. **Voluntary agreement:** The participation has to be voluntary without any force or coercion.

Several things need to be taken into account for a complete informed consent document (Table 10.5).

Writing a good informed consent is a balancing act between being thorough, being accurate, and being as concise and simple as possible. Also the patient advocates may offer invaluable experience and insight during the drafting and review phase of an informed consent in clinical trials.

Table 10.5: Components of informed consent

- Be thorough and complete
- Simple, nontechnical language
- Carefully worded to avoid potentially coercive phrasing
- Statement that the study involves research
- Purpose of the research and the length of the study
- Contains description of risks and benefits
- Discussion of alternative therapies
- Confidentiality policy
- Compensation for injury
- Contact for further questions/information
- Statement of voluntary participation

Endpoints in Research Protocol

Endpoints in research protocol are the identifiable change that shows the intervention did what it was supposed to do. They can be primary or surrogate (secondary).

Primary endpoints measure the specific clinical effect the intervention is preventing/treating (i.e. survival, resolution of disease, subjective well-being, etc).

Surrogate endpoints measure changes in symptom/biological indicator for the success of the intervention (i.e. blood cell count, radiographic imaging, etc.)

Study Schedule

Methodology and study schedule should be described in detail. A brief overview is given in Table 10.6.

Table 10.6: Study schedule

- Description of recruitment and enrollment procedures
- Screening and allocation of subjects
- Subject numbering system
- Preparation of study drug for use
- Schedule for administration of test article to subject
- Contraindications
- Schedule of visits and assessments
- Measures to maintain blinding/unblinding procedures
- Required documentation

Measurements in Research

At each and every stage, the study measures and assessments along with the detailed technique should be mentioned like:

- Physical examinations
- Measurements of vital signs
- Assessment procedures
- Clinical laboratory
- Handling of samples
- Special safety requirements.

Detailed description of study procedures/interventions have to be given. This needs the research procedures described in detail so they can be performed consistently. The intervention should be detailed but not the common medical procedures like blood pressure/sugar measurement, etc. These may not need detail. Procedures for carrying out physical exams, vital signs, handling samples may be very detailed if it is essential to the data collection.

Laboratory Details

Laboratory procedure need to be explained in detail specially if it involves collection of biological samples, e.g. blood. For example, the Protocol states 10 ml of blood; then one should explain why this much amount and why not less, etc. Additionally, several questions need to be answered. Mostly the reviewers will emphasize the necessarily to take lesser amount of blood samples (Table 10.7).

Statistics

Make sure that study objectives and study design elements in the statistical section mirror those in described in the objectives section. If the study involves stopping rules, make sure that descriptions and definitions of toxicities

Table 10.7: Questions about the laboratory procedures

- What tubes are needed to draw samples?
- What is the minimum amount of blood needed?
- Does the sample need to be on ice?
- Does it need to be processed same day?
- Sample needs storage?

in the statistical section match those in the safety/adverse event section.

Prevent Errors

Many existing clinical trials contain problems, such as incompleteness, ambiguity, and inconsistency. Most of the errors are introduced during the protocol writing process. This has to be guarded against. Costs of a badly written protocol can lead to rejection. To fix this problem, the protocol has to be amended. Remember any change to the protocol document or informed consent that affects the scientific intent, study design, patient safety, or human subject protection is considered an amendment, and therefore *must* be approved by your institutional review board. To be able to prevent errors, fresh eyes are needed. Working too long on a protocol may habituate eyes and brains to mistakes, simply because they have been there all along. That means, one would have get an "outside" reviewer. Simple things such as spell-checkers, etc. should be kept in mind. One should remember that a document that has been "checked" by automatic software has not been proofread. Poorly written inclusion criteria have resulted in a number of ineligible and invaluable patients being enrolled to a study.

Protocol Evaluation

This is usually done by institute review board with an aim to ensure subject protection. The funding agencies like National Institute of Health, Indian Council of Medical Research too evaluate protocols. Sometimes regulatory agencies like Food and Drug Administration (Drug Controller General of India) too overview the protocol. The aim is to protect public health. Investigator himself/herself has to see the feasibility, scientific interest and other details of the study. Study coordinator will have to see operational implementation of the study. Finally protocol should be made in such a way that it goes through the IRB review. To be able to achieve that one should ask himself/herselves that if the protocol is scientifically valid? The safety, and the risk/benefit ratio, ethical issues will have to be evaluated thoroughly.

Bibliography

1. Office of Human Subjects Research http://ohsr.od.nih.gov/info/info.html/
2. Protomechanics: http://www.cc.nih.gov/ccc/protomechanics
3. The Cancer Therapy Evaluation Program (CTEP) Templates (phases I–III; based on NIH model): http://ctep.cancer.gov/guidelines/templates.html
4. The International Committee of Medical Journal Editors (ICJME) Uniform Requirements for Manuscripts Submitted to Biomedical Journals http://www.icmje.org/
5. The NCI Investigators' Handbook: http://ctep.cancer.gov/handbook/index.html
6. The NIH phase III template: http://www.ninds. nih.gov/funding/research/clinical_research/ProtocolTemplate.htm
7. The Office for Human Research Protections (OHRP): http://www.hhs.gov/ohrp/policy/index.html#informed
8. The Office of Human Subjects Research: http://ohsr.od.nih.gov/info/info.html

Review of Literature

Learning objectives

This chapter starts with what is a literature review and why the review the literature is done? One has to plan the search by putting appropriate keywords or using the joint or Boolean search. One can easily use snowballing/tracking citations. Additionally, one would have to choose appropriate databases or sources to search the needed items.

What is a Literature Review?

A literature review by definition "is a systematic method for identifying, evaluating and interpreting the work produced by researchers, scholars and practitioners".

This should not be a random process but a systematically coordinated search to look for what do we want. In the beginning, students search hours if not days or months to search for the topic of interest. In MSc/MD/PhD for initial few months, this is an activity that lasts for long-time.

Why do we Review Literature?

This is like knowing the address of a person whom we want to have a meeting. Naturally, without good literature review, one would not acquire an understanding of the topic, of what has already been done on it, how it has been researched, and what the key issues are. So this not only does serve the purpose of knowing the topic in-depth, but also helps us knowing the key lacunas.

Getting Started

Nowadays, getting started with literature review is easy. In the gone by era, it used to take lot of time as one would have search through voluminous books and printed journals. Nowadays, it is done via internet and there are dozens of handy sources to know the literature in-depth. One can start with the broad problem area but do not be too global (e.g. searching the history of medicine when the topic is on specifically upon "history of psychopharmacology"). By changing one keywords, the search strategy changes and one would end up getting hundreds of different articles. Broad rules of search the literature are given in Table 11.1.

Table 11.1: Do's and Don'ts in literature search	
Do	*Don't*
Define search term, and be specific	Cover everything in your area of interest and keeping the search term very broad
Pick-up most relevant articles	Trying to read everything in a short span of time
Focus on the search question	Trying to get a hang of lot of things and then narrow down on the search term

Guidelines to Medical Literature Search in Research

When starting, it is important to cover research relevant to all the variables being studied. Also, the research that explains the relationship between these variables is a top priority rather than being general and trying to search too much too soon. One would need to plan how the structure his/her literature review will appear and write from his/her plan and follow the same. While doing the literature search several issues may come up and need to be addressed (Table 11.2).

Table 11.2: Issues to consider when searching medical literature

- Use right keywords to search
- Narrowing the search as much as possible
- Using the library effectively
- Search only relevant articles
- Read articles intended for particular audience
- Search latest information
- Look for coverage of the topic of interest
- Accuracy of the information provided
- Authority of the author or information source
- Level of objectivity of the author
- Clarity of information provided

Organized Search

It is important to know the topic one is searching and be organized about the same and search for related articles for the snowballing effect. Following is a useful way of being organized.

a. **Topical order:** One can organize by main topics or issues; emphasize the relationship of the issues to the main "problem". For example, searching "Yoga and Rheumatoid arthritis " is much better than searching for "Yoga and Health".

b. **Chronological order:** One can organize the literature by the dates the research was published.

c. **Problem-cause-solution order:** One can organize the review so that it moves from the problem to the solution. For example, "hypertension and drug therapy" is a better keyword rather than "drugs and hypertension".

d. **Funnel approach:** This is like being "General to specific search. One can examine broad-based research first and then focus on specific studies that relate to the topic. For example, going for neurology, to dementia, to Alzheimer's disease, to beta-amyloid to anti-beta-amyloid vaccine/adverse effects of vaccine, etc.

e. **Lacuna order:** After reviewing the literature, summarize what has been done, what has not been done, and what needs to be done. One can easily make such notes.

Good Literature Review

Good medical literature review done for research purposes is a critical assay that assess range of medical literature available and can always yield surprising results. A reviewer is supposed to have the critical attitude and one should not take the published medical literature at face value and be able to question the same as well. A good review should go beyond simply listing relevant literature (i.e. helpful in understanding state-of-art information on the subject of interest). Additional features of a good review are given in Table 11.3.

Table 11.3: Features of good literature review

- Is a critical essay (critical summary)
- Assesses the range of literature available
- Examines the background against which research is set
- Forms a significant section of thesis
- Relates different writings to each other, compares and contrasts available studies
- Uses particular language: authors assert, argue, state, conclude, etc.
- Shows an awareness of the theories and values that underlie the research

Defining Search

One has to use an appropriate keyword/s. A good review is all about the same. If the key-words chosen are different, then one will find it hard to do the same. One would have to identify the significant terms and concepts that describe topic from the point of view of thesis or research question. Remember, once the work you do gets published, these terms will become the key for searching catalogs, databases and search engines for information about your subject. Then the rules that we have talked about in this chapter will be read by students and the cycle gets repeated.

Boolean

- And = Narrow
- Not = Exclude

- Or = Expand

Snowballing

Building on the works of others and one related article will give link to the another. A scholarly article will always have references/ bibliography. A bibliography is always ripe for the picking by the next interested reader.

Choosing Databases

One should choose appropriate databases. It should be noted that Google is not (usually) the best answer. Also, without criticizing, Wikipedia is also not a great idea that students come up with. One should start with library resources for your subject first. Then search a range of databases and think about the range of sources: books, journal articles, statistics, websites, conference reports, etc. for good literature search. Examples of some of the commonly used databases are given in Table 11.4.

Table 11.4: Examples of some databases
• Academic search complete
• Psycharticles
• SocIndex with full text
• TOPIC search
• Web MD

Search Method

One can start by creating a folder and then try and narrow the research. Scholarly journals publications can be filtered by publication dates, subject, thesaurus terms, etc.

Google Scholar

Google scholar (Fig. 11.1) is a very popular database and provides a simple way to search for scholarly literature. One can search books, abstracts and articles, from academic publishers, professional societies, preprint repositories, universities and other scholarly organizations. Such a simple search tool works best for citations. However, some full text articles may be have restrictions to the content and may be fee-based. One can contact the library if they have the subscription. Other common databases are MSN (www.msn.com), yahoo (www.yahoo.com) and bing (www.bing.com).

Fig. 11.1: Search engines like google are instant source of useful information. However, whatever we get in this search engine should not be taken blindly as the information can be written by non professionals also. So the obtained information should be credible

Common Errors in Literature Review

Review may not be logically organized and this is a common error. Also it may not be focused on most important facets of the study. The worse is when the review does not relate literature to the study. There may be too few references or outdated references cited. Review is not written in author's own words and may be a cut and paste material. Review reads like a series of disjointed summaries and this can distract them easily. Review that does not argue a point and hence may not be balanced; recent references may have been omitted.

Plagiarism

Plagiarism includes using another writer's words without proper citation. Also the use of another writer's ideas without proper citation constitutes plagiarism. Citing a source but reproducing the exact word without quotation marks could also be plagiarism. Borrowing the structure of another author's phrases/sentences without giving the source. Borrowing all or part of another student's paper could be a simple yet serious form of plagiarism. Using paper-writing service or having a friend write the paper is a cheating (Fig. 11.2).

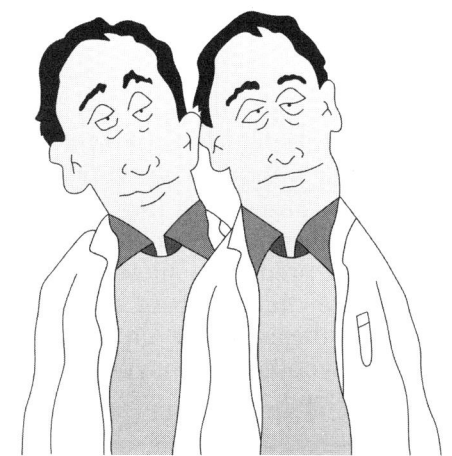

Fig. 11.2: Copy and paste can seriously jeopardize the review

After Literature Search

After the search is completed, the one has to argue the point as to why is the study is important. Then one can pose a formal research question or state a hypothesis and this has to be linked to the literature review. All sources cited in the literature review should be listed in the references as well. To sum, a literature review should include introduction, summary and critique of journal articles, justifications for the research project and the hypothesis for the research project. Individual components described here have been discussed at length in individual chapters as well.

Bibliography

1. How to do literature review? www.faculty. swosu.edu/frederic.murray/DunnLit Review. ppt (Accessed online on July 14th 2016).
2. How to write a literature review. http:// library.bcu.ac.uk/learner/writingguides/ 1.04.htm (Accessed online on January 31st 2017).
3. Literature Reviews: An Overview for Graduate Students.https://www.lib.ncsu.edu/ tutorials/ litreview/(Accessed online on January 31st 2017).Subjects Research: http:// ohsr.od.nih.gov/info/info.html
4. The University of North Carolina. http:// writingcenter.unc.edu/handouts/literature- reviews/(Accessed online on January 31st 2017).
5. University of California. http://guides. library.ucsc.edu/write-a-literature-review. (Accessed online on January 31st 2017).

Bias and Errors

Learning objectives

Error is the difference between the true value of a measurement and the recorded value. For example, a good instrument which is well-calibrated gives blood pressure recording of an adult male patient as 120/80 mm Hg while the other one gives 140/90; there is error in the 2nd instrument. There could be several sources of errors in clinical data collections and can be random or systematic. Random error is something that is hard to detect and occurs by chance hence is also called variability, random variation, or 'noise in the system'.

What is an error?

An error generally defined as the false or mistaken result obtained in a study or experiment. Errors are of two main types: *random* and *systematic* error (Fig. 12.1).

Random error is the portion of variation in measurement that has no apparent connection to any other measurement or variable, generally regarded as due to chance. *Systematic error* which often has a recognizable source, e.g. a faulty measuring instrument, or pattern, e.g. it is consistently wrong in a particular direction.

Hypothesis

All analytic studies must begin with a clearly formulated hypothesis. The hypothesis must be *quantitative* and *specific* (Fig. 12.2). It must predict a relationship of a specific size. Only specific prediction allows one to draw legitimate conclusions from a study which tests a hypothesis. But even with the best formulated hypothesis, two types of errors can occur (*see* below).

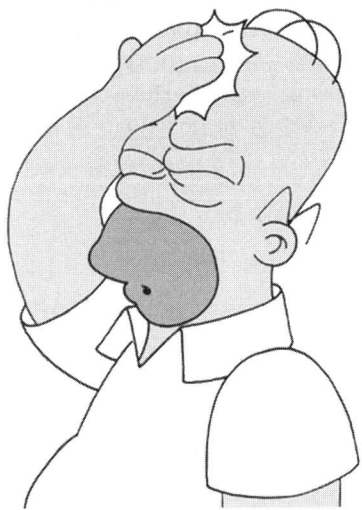

Fig. 12.1: Errors in research are common and unless fixed or accounted for, they can reduce internal and external validity

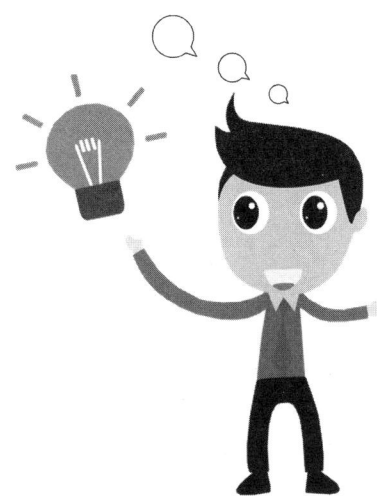

Fig. 12.2: Hypothesis is a testable idea based upon sound theory/scientific facts

Type 1: These types of errors are said to be present when someone is observing a difference when in truth there is none. These types of errors can bring about misleading consequences and could be serious. The most serious result is the introduction of a drug that did not have the potential to treat!

Type 2: Type 2 errors are little less serious but surely, will have consequences. These errors arise when the observer fails to observe a difference when there is one. This is like someone is unable to spot the difference.

These errors are generally produced by one or more of the following:

  a. Random errors
  b. Random classification
  c. Bias
  d. Confounding

Hence, it is important to review these terms in detail.

Random Error

Random error is the deviation of results and inferences from the truth, occurring only as a result of the operation of chance. It can produce type 1 or type 2 errors. Random error could due to the measurement of an exposure or outcome. A random error can also occur due to measuring instrument or changes in surrounding. For example, we wish to measure weights of 1st year college students of a given college. The weighing machine that day may have been placed on uneven surface and hence, the results will show variations from the true values.

Clarification Error

Errors in classification can only produce type 2 errors, except if applied to *a confounder* or to an *exposure gradient.*

Bias

Bias is a systematic, non-random deviation of results and inferences from the truth, or processes (e.g. repeatedly wrong measurement of blood pressure) leading to such deviation. Peculiar trend in the collection, analysis,

interpretation, publication or review of data can lead to conclusions which are systematically different from the truth need to be watched out for to avoid such a conclusion.

Note that in bias, the focus is on an *artifact* of some part of the research *process* (assembling subjects, collecting data, analyzing data) that produces a spurious result. Bias can produce either a type 1 or a type 2 error, but we usually focus on type 1 errors due to bias.

Bias can be either conscious or unconscious: In epidemiology, the word bias does not imply, as in common usage, prejudice or deliberate deviation from the truth. Deviation of results or inferences from the truth, or processes leading to such deviation can distort scientific results. Hence, any trend in the collection, analysis, interpretation, publication, or review of data that can lead to conclusions that are systematically different from the truth. In summary, *bias may be understood as a process at any stage of inference tending to produce results that depart systematically from true values.*

1. SELECTION BIAS

Any aspect of the *way subjects are assembled in the study* that creates a systematic difference between the compared populations that is not due to the association under study. Selection bias can lead to errors due to systematic differences in characteristics between those who are selected for study and those who are not. When comparisons are made between groups of patients that differ in ways other than the main factors under study, outcome under study gets affected.

2. INFORMATION BIAS

Any aspect of the *way information is collected in the study* that creates a systematic difference between the compared populations that is not due to the factors under study (some call this measurement bias). The incomplete chart recording in the baby feeding example would be a form of information bias (Fig. 12.3).

Other example of such bias can be diagnostic bias or recall bias. Sometimes biases apply to a population of studies, rather than to one

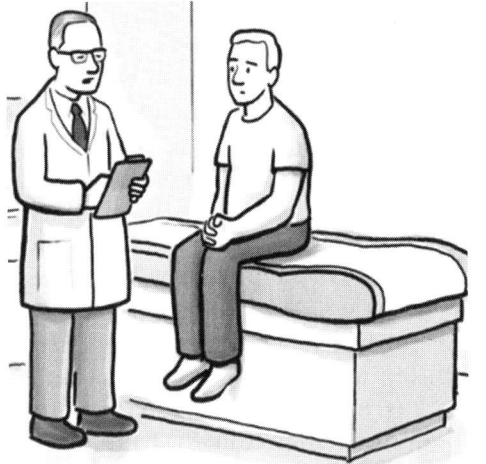

Fig. 12.3: Method of information collection in the study has to be uniform otherwise information bias could be a problem

study, as in publication bias (tendency to publish papers which show positive results).

Ascertainment Bias

Systematic failure to represent equally all classes of cases or persons supposed to be represented in a sample. This bias may arise because of the nature of the sources from which the persons come, e.g. a specialized clinic; from a diagnostic process influenced by culture, custom, or idiosyncrasy (Fig. 12.4).

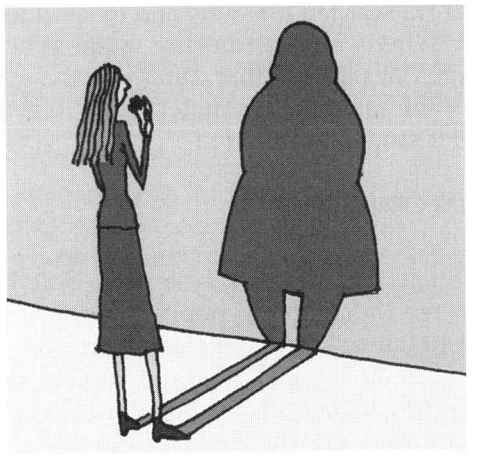

Fig. 12.4: Ascertainment bias can be due to distorted results. It can seriously jeopardize the generalization of study

Response bias is a systematic error due to differences in characteristics between those who choose or volunteer to take part in a study and those who do not. Volunteers may drop-out either because they are unwell, or worried about an exposure.

Susceptibility Bias

Groups being compared are not equally susceptible to the outcome of interest, for reasons other than the factors under study. It is comparable to 'Assembly Bias'. In prognosis studies; cohorts may differ in one or more ways—extent of disease, presence of other diseases, the point of time in the course of disease, prior treatment, etc. (Fig. 12.5).

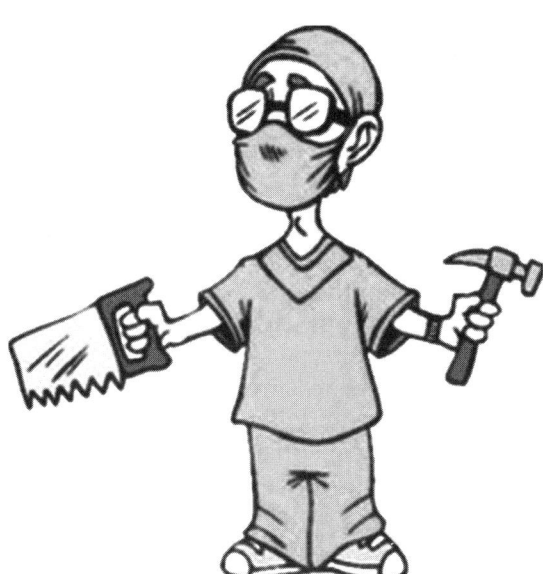

Fig. 12.5: Some patients are susceptible to respond to one form of treatment compared to the other, e.g. those who received surgery will respond better compared to chemotherapy

Migration Bias

In nearly all large studies some members of the original cohort dropout of the study. If dropouts occur randomly, such that characteristics of lost subjects in one group are on an average similar to those who remain in the group, no bias is introduced. But ordinarily the characteristics of the lost subjects are not the same (Fig. 12.6).

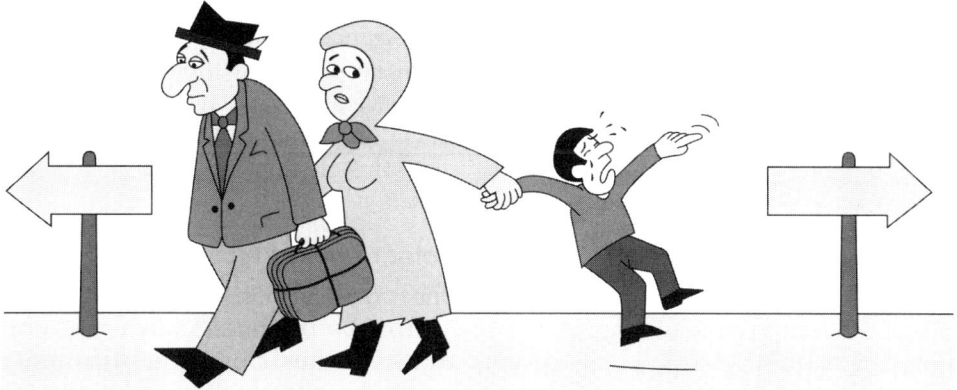

Fig. 12.6: Migration of some of the patients in cohort studies can create bias

Healthy Worker Bias

Last defines healthy worker bias as a phenomenon observed initially in studies of occupational diseases: workers usually exhibit lower overall death rates than the general population, because the severely ill and chronically disabled are ordinarily excluded from employment. Death rates in the general population may be inappropriate for comparison if this effect is not taken into account.

Measurement Bias

As per last, systematic error arising from inaccurate measurements (or classification) of subjects or study variables. It occurs when individual measurements or classifications of disease or exposure are inaccurate (i.e. they do not measure correctly what they are supposed to measure). If patients in one group stand a better chance of having their outcomes detected than those in another group.

Hawthorne Effect

This effect which is usually positive/beneficial of being under study upon the persons being studied; their knowledge of being studied influences their behavior.

Placebo Effect

This is usually, but not necessarily beneficial expectation that regimen will have effect, i.e. the effect is due to the power of suggestion.

Misclassification Bias

This could be of several varieties, e.g. exposure misclassification occurs when exposed subjects are incorrectly classified as unexposed, or vice versa. Disease misclassification occurs when diseased subjects are incorrectly classified as non-diseased, or vice versa. Measurement gap is a gap between the measured and the true value of a variable. It may suffer from the following:

- Observer/interviewer bias
- Recall bias
- Reporting bias

The gap between the theoretical and empirical definition of exposure/disease.

Confounding

A problem resulting from the fact that one feature of study subjects *has not been separated* from a second feature, and has thus been *confounded* with it, producing a spurious result. The spuriousness arises from the effect of the first feature being mistakenly attributed to the second feature. Confounding can produce either a type 1 or a type 2 error, but we usually focus on type 1 errors. So basically, confounding is a situation in which the effects of two processes are not separated. The distortion of the apparent effect of an exposure on risk brought about by the association with other factors that can influence the outcome. This is a relationship between the effects of two or more causal factors as observed in a set of data such that it is not logically possible to separate the contribution that any single causal factor has made to an effect. Last defines confounding as a situation when another exposure exists in the study population (besides the one being studied) and is associated both with disease and the exposure being studied. If this extraneous factor—itself a determinant of or risk factor for health outcome is unequally distributed between the exposure subgroups, it can lead to confounding.

In summary, confounder is a risk factor among the unexposed (itself a determinant of disease). It is associated with the exposure under study and is unequally distributed among the exposed and the unexposed groups.

Difference between Bias and Confounding

Bias creates an association that is not true, but confounding describes an association that is true, but potentially misleading. The factor that creates the bias, or the confounding variable, *must be associated with both the independent and dependent variables* (i.e. with the exposure and the disease). Association of the bias or confounder with just one of the two variables is not enough to produce a spurious result. Were the bias or the confounder associated with *just* the independent variable or *just* the dependent variable, they would not produce bias or confounding. This gives a useful rule: If you can show that a potential confounder is NOT associated with either one of the two variables under study (exposure or outcome), confounding can be ruled out.

How to Protect Against Random Error?

Random error can work to falsely produce an association (type 1 error) or falsely not produce an association (type 2 error). We protect ourselves against random misclassification producing a type 2 error by choosing the most *precise and accurate* measures of exposure and outcome.

Protect Against Type 1 Errors

We protect our study against random type 1 errors by establishing that the result must be unlikely to have occurred by chance (e.g. p < .05). *P-values* are established entirely to protect against type 1 errors due to chance, and *do not guarantee protection against type 1 errors due to bias or confounding.* This is the reason we say statistics demonstrate *association* but not *causation.*

Protect Against Type 2 Errors

One can protect the study against random type 2 errors by providing adequate sample size, and hypothesizing large differences. The larger the sample size, the easier it will be to detect a true difference, and the largest differences will be the easiest to detect.

How to Increase Study Power?

The sample size needed to detect a significant difference is called the *power* of a study. Choosing the most *precise and accurate* measures of exposure and outcome has the effect of increasing the power of our study, because of variances of the outcome measures, which enter into statistical testing, are decreased. Having an adequate sized sample of study subjects.

Matching

As per last, it is a process of making a study group and a comparison group comparable with respect to extraneous factors. For each patient in one group there are one or more patients in the comparison group with same characteristics, except for the factor of interest. Matching may be of several types:

a. **Caliper matching:** This is a process of matching comparison group to study group within a specific distance for a continuous variable (e.g. matching age to within 2 years).

b. **Frequency matching:** This involves frequency distributions of the matched variable be similar in study and comparison groups.

c. **Category matching:** This type of matching the groups in broad classes, such as relatively wide age ranges or occupational groups.

d. **Individual matching:** This is a process involving identification of individual subjects for comparison, each resembling a study subject on the matched variable(s).

e. **Pair matching:** Individual matching in which the study and comparison subjects are paired.

Matching is often done for age, sex, race, place of residence, severity of disease, rate of progression of disease, previous treatment received, etc. The limitations of matching involves controls for bias for only those factors involved in the match. Also, it is usually not possible to match for more than a few factors because of the practical difficulties of finding patients that meet all matching criteria. If categories for matching are relatively crude, there may be room for substantial differences between matched groups.

Overmatching

Overmatching may occur if the matching variable is involved in, or is closely connected with, the mechanism whereby the independent variable affects the dependant variable. The matching variable may be an intermediate cause in the causal chain or it may be strongly affected by, or a consequence of, such an intermediate cause.

Stratification

Stratification is the process of or the result of separating a sample into several sub-samples according to specified criteria, such as age groups, socio-economic status, etc. he effect of confounding variables may be controlled by stratifying the analysis of results. It is important to know that after the data are collected, they can be analyzed and results presented according to subgroups of patients, or strata, of similar characteristics.

Standardization

Standardization is a set of techniques used to remove as far as possible the effects of differences in age or other confounding variables when comparing two or more populations. This is a method that uses weighted averaging of rates specific for age, sex, or some other potentially confounding variable(s), according to some specified distribution of these variables. Direct standardization involves the specific rates in a study population are averaged using as weights the distribution of a specified standard population.

Standardization vs Stratification

Standardization removes the effect but stratification controls for the effect of factor, but the effect can still be seen, e.g. in the 'hospital example', with standardization we found that patients had similar prognosis in both hospitals; with stratification also learnt mortality rates among different risk strata. Similar to difference between age-standardized mortality rate and age specific mortality rates could be found. It needs to be known that a good study design protects against all forms of errors.

Bibliography

1. Bias and error. http://conflict.lshtm.ac.uk/page_40.htm (Downloaded May 3rd 2017).
2. Bias and systematic errors. https://www.ctspedia.org/do/view/CTSpedia/Bias Definition (Downloaded May 3rd 2017).
3. Understanding bias and errors. http://scott.fortmann-roe.com/docs/BiasVariance.html (Downloaded May 3rd 2017).

Diagnostic Testing in Basic and Clinical Epidemiology

Learning objectives

Patients present with symptoms, and are suspected of having some disease. One of the important aims of doctors is to determine whether the patients either have the disease or do not have the disease. Physician performs a diagnostic test to assist in making a diagnosis. The test result is either positive (diseased) or negative (healthy). A given test has two important objectives: to distinguish between people in the population who have the diseases and those who do not. The diagnostic testing is done primarily to determine how good the test is in separating populations of people with and without the disease in question?

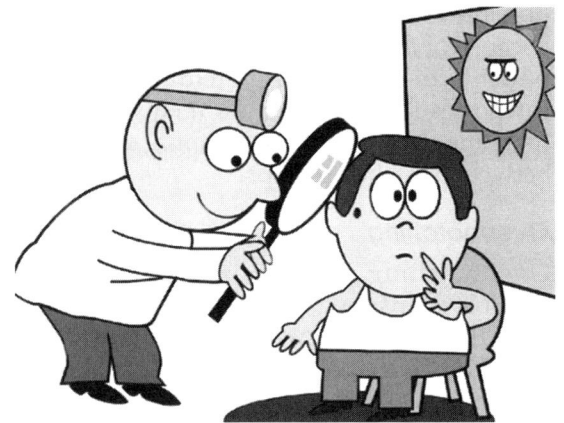

Fig. 13.1: Screening tests are used for diagnosis and prognostication. One should be aware about their ability to detect the disease (sensitivity) and to separate healthy from disease (specificity)

SCREENING TEST

A screening test should have sensitivity, specificity, predictive value, validity and precision. Sensitivity is the probability that a person who truly has the disease correctly receives a positive test result, while the specificity is the probability that a person who is truly healthy correctly receives a negative test result. It goes without saying that the ones who are healthy should not be labeled with disease and the ones who do have the disease should be diagnosed by the diagnostic test (Fig. 13.1).

Use of Screening Tests

Screening tests are used in medical diagnosis, screening, and research. We use medical tests to diagnose health conditions. Positive test results can have profound effects on human beings (e.g. positive hepatitis B, HIV positive). Yet no test is infallible and both false positive and negatives do occur.

False positive results means the healthy person incorrectly receives a positive (diseased) test result. For example, someone who had sexual exposure was sent to HIV testing lab and the result was given as wrongly positive. False negative result means that the diseased person incorrectly receives a negative (healthy) test result.

One should minimize the chance or probability of false positive and false negative test results. Or, alternatively, maximize probability of correct results (Fig. 13.2).

Why do Diagnostic Test

Diagnostic testing is done to reduce uncertainty regarding a specific patient's diagnosis. Generally diagnostic testing is most appropriate in the presence of intermediate (10 to 90%)

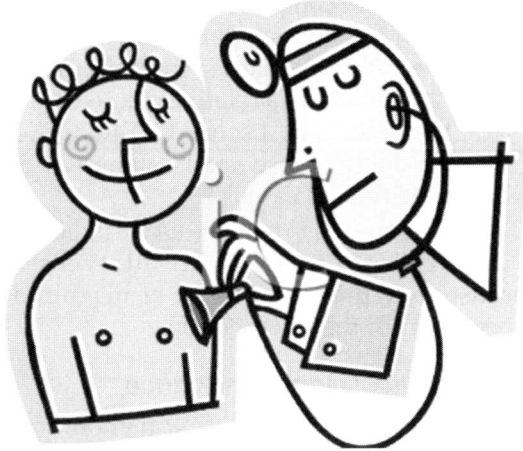

Fig. 13.2: Diagnostic tests may have the probability of being false positive (reduced sensitivity) and false negative (reduced specificity)

pretest probability of a disease. This is determined by the clinical diagnosis. Test characteristics (i.e. likelihood ratios) should be considered before ordering a test to help determine whether a given test would significantly change post-test probability (and thus affect management). Diagnostic tests should only be used if the result is likely to significantly affect certainty of a disease (post-test probability) and should rely on likelihood ratios for a given test when available. It is important to know that we have used the terms "pretest" and "post-test" here; the former refers to sensitivity and specificity while the latter refers to positive and negative predictive value.

An Overview of Diagnostic Tests

Major goal of screening are to detect treatable, asymptomatic, or early stage disease. The limitations, harms, and costs associated with screening should be considered in the context of the patient's goals. Whenever possible, treatment benefit should be expressed in terms of absolute risk reduction (not relative risk reduction).

Likelihood Ratio

Likelihood ratios (LRs) combine the sensitivity and specificity of a test with pretest probability

of disease in a specific patient, avoiding the need to perform statistical calculations based on test characteristics and prevalence data.

$$LR+ = \text{sensitivity}/(1-\text{specificity})$$

$$LR- = (1-\text{sensitivity})/\text{specificity}$$

They provide a sense of how "powerful" a test is in influencing our pretest probability of disease. Likelihood ratios may be positive [LR(+)], which are used when assessing for the presence of disease when a test result is positive, and negative [LR(–)], which are used when excluding disease with a negative test result.

Likelihood ratios may also be calculated sequentially with serial testing, if needed. To detect asymptomatic and early stage disease. The test should be highly sensitive and highly specific to pick up most cases of true disease and avoid false positives. The test should be targeted toward populations with a higher disease prevalence (high positive predictive value). Should be relatively safe and cost-effective. The test should screen for diseases in which early identification and treatment have been demonstrated to improve clinical outcomes.

False Positive

False positive results can occur in tests. The primary goal of screening is to find specific diseases—maximize sensitivity at cost of specificity and this may lead to—false positives. This can lead to incorrect labelling, inconvenience, expense, and physical harm in follow-up tests.

Predictive value

$$\text{Positive PV} = \frac{\text{True positives}}{\text{TP + FP}} \times 100 = \%$$

$$\text{Negative PV} = \frac{\text{True negatives}}{\text{TN + FN}} \times 100 = \%$$

Limitations of Screening

Screening is a useful tool to detect diseases but the lead time bias can make diagnosis of disease earlier! This may ensure false survival benefits! Length time bias can lead to over-diagnosis and pseudodisease can emerge.

Hence, it is recommended that one should screen less frequently. Also one should not screen patients with a life expectancy less than 10 years. One should discuss potential downstream testing with patient before ordering initial screening test. Also, one can use higher threshold for positive result. Understand basic test characteristics and limitations, as well as an individual patient's goals and values.

Absolute Risk (AR)

Absolute Risk (AR) or Event Rate (ER) is the probability of an event occurring in a group during a specified time period. Patients with event in group/total patients in group.

Relative Risk (RR)

Relative risk is the ratio of the probability of developing a disease with a risk factor present to the probability of developing the disease without the risk factor present.

Absolute Risk Reduction (ARR)

Absolute risk reduction is the difference in rates of events between experimental group and control group, i.e. Experimental Event Rate (EER) and Control Event Rate (CER).

Relative Risk Reduction (RRR)

Relative risk reduction is the ratio of absolute risk reduction to the event rate among controls, i.e. experimental event rate and control event rate/control event rate.

Number Needed to Treat (NNT)

Number needed to treat is the number of patients needed to receive a treatment for one additional patient to benefit.

This is calculated by = 1/absolute risk reduction.

Number Needed to Harm (NNH)

Number needed to harm is the number of patients needed to receive a treatment for one additional patient to be harmed. This is calculated by = 1/absolute risk increase.

One should use absolute risk, absolute risk reduction, and numbers needed whenever

possible. Relative comparisons may exaggerate uncommon outcomes. Interventions that reduce the rate of a disease from 40 to 20% and 4 to 2% each have a relative risk reduction of 50%. However, the Absolute Risk Reduction (ARR) for the first case is 20%, whereas the ARR for the second case is 2%.

Numbers needed to treat are useful indicators of the clinical impact of an intervention because they provide a sense of magnitude expected from the intervention.

Statistical vs Clinical Significance

Statistical significance and clinical importance are intimately linked and this is a common question. Especially for large studies with uncommon outcomes; this question is especially relevant (Fig. 13.3).

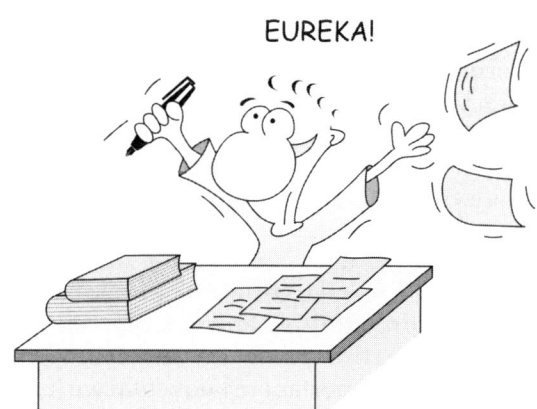

Fig. 13.3: Something that is statistically significant may not have clinical significance. It is important to know that the latter is more important

True disease status	Test result	
	Diseased (+)	Healthy (−)
Diseased (+)	Correct	False negative
Healthy (−)	False positive	Correct

Clinical Epidemiology

Clinical epidemiology deals with the application of the principles and methods of epidemiology to clinical practice. This is a relatively new kid on the block of epidemiology and hence is continuously evolving.

This is a basic science and its popularity in medical colleges is growing. Since India is a projected hub of clinical research worldwide, this is supposed to grow even more in India.

Clinical Epidemiology as a Contraindication

Some would assume that epidemiology deals with population and clinical epidemiology deals with individuals. Therefore, is it a sort of contraindication?

Principles and practice of clinical epidemiology could be applied to a localized population and hence, this conflict could easily be resolved (Fig. 13.4) .

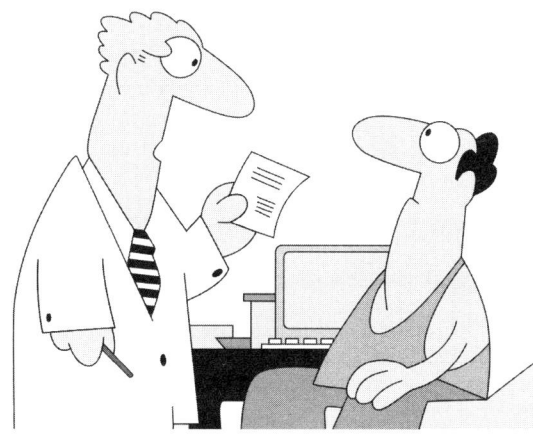

Fig. 13.4: Clinical epidemiology lays down principles that can be applied in a group of people so that by using them the group gets benefited unlike clinical medicine that is focused on the individual

Importance of Clinical Epidemiology

One could easily question the importance of epidemiology as a discipline in clinics. However, it could:

a. Help doctors, nurses, pharmacists and physiotherapists to improve clinical practice.

b. To be able to recommend to health authorities about any information that could be generated and improve health situation further.

It is said that clinical epidemiology training and understanding is essential for practice

clinically for doctors and nurses; expertise in this discipline of epidemiology could differ.

Main Concerns in Clinical Epidemiology

Following are the main concerns:
- What is normal?
- What is abnormal?
- Diagnostic accuracy
- Natural history
- Predicting prognosis
- Effectiveness of treatment
- Prevention in clinical practice.

Define Normality and Abnormality

Clinically, it is very important to know what is normal or abnormal? So practically, clinicians need to know workable definitions of disease.

Two-standard deviations above or below means: This is a popular definition of what is normal or abnormal in clinical epidemiology. If the population follows normal distribution (also called Gaussian distribution); then 2.5% of the population will be classified as abnormal (Fig. 13.5).

Ninety-five (95%) percentile as a definition: A 95% percentile definition also exists and assumes that 95% of the population is normal and rest of them (5%) are abnormal.

Limitation of this definition is that for most of "cut-offs", there is no biological variable that could be chosen to define them. Like, e.g. nomograms are yet to be developed for how much of increase in blood pressure will contribute to how much increase in cerebrovascular accidents.

Abnormal as "Diseased"

A clear separation in epidemiology between normal and abnormal is needed for us to be able to workout with people and populations (Table 13.1).

Unfortunately in epidemiology, separating abnormal from normal is difficult. This will mean, some "cases" could always be found in "normal".

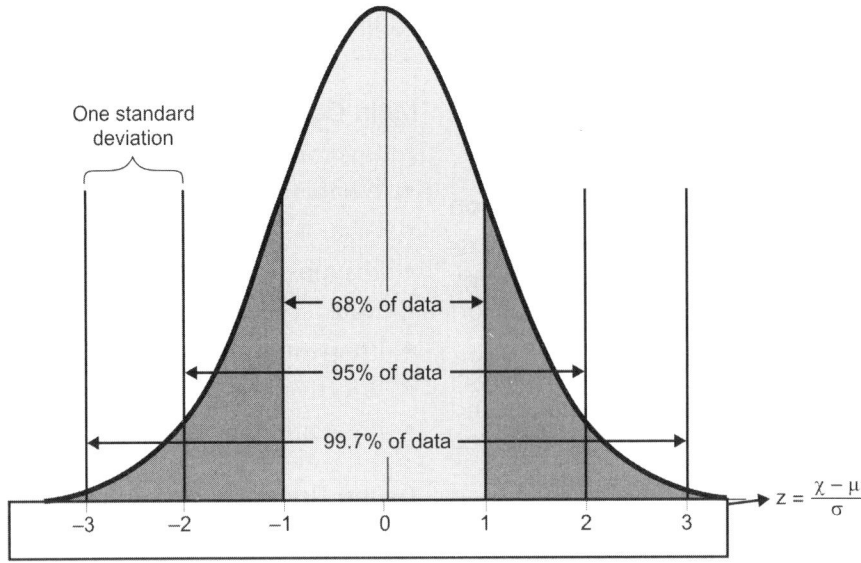

Fig. 13.5: Majority of the data is centred around the mean in normal distribution

Sensitivity and specificity

Sensitivity: Ability of a diagnostic test to be able to pick up true positive cases reflects sensitivity.

Specificity: Ability of a diagnostic rest to be able to pick up true negative (healthy case) is called specificity.

Clearly, a disease may be present or absent. But one can also however have true positive, false positive, true negative and false negative combinations. Such combinations are very important in diagnostic testing as these could tell us whether a given test will be able to predict the disease occurrence with confidence or not.

Both sensitivity and specificity in epidemiology need to be handled with care (Figs 13.6 and 13.7).

Increase in one could lead to decrease in other (Fig. 13.8).

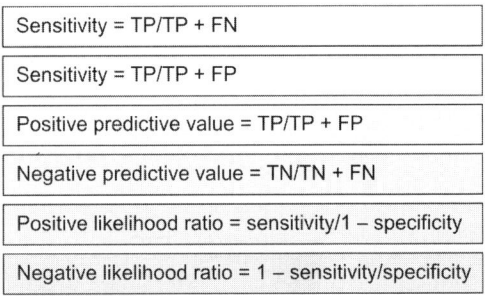

Sensitivity = TP/TP + FN
Sensitivity = TP/TP + FP
Positive predictive value = TP/TP + FP
Negative predictive value = TN/TN + FN
Positive likelihood ratio = sensitivity/1 – specificity
Negative likelihood ratio = 1 – sensitivity/specificity

Fig. 13.6: Commonly used formulas in diagnostic testing

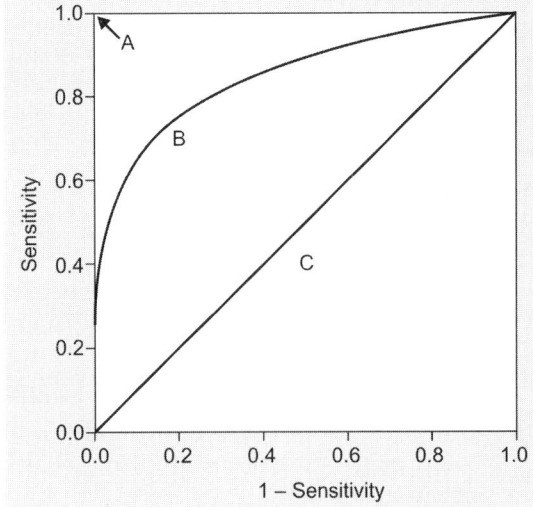

Table 13.1: Diagnostic test and disease occurrence (e.g. VDRL in dementia)

Diagnostic test	Positive	True positive	False positive
	Negative	False negative	True negative

*VDRL = Venereal disease research laboratory

Fig. 13.7: Receiver Operating Characteristic (ROC) curve. Note the relationship between sensitivity and specificity

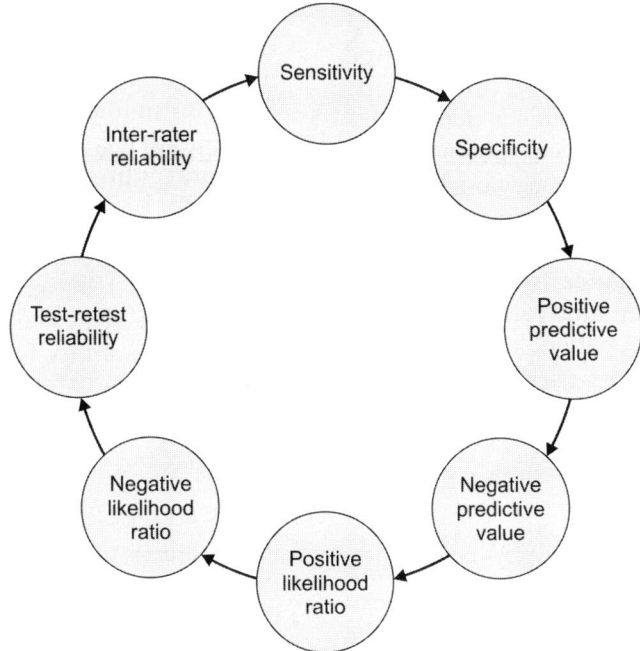

Fig. 13.8: Almost all the parameters of diagnostic testing are inter-related with each other

Both are affected by prevalence and low prevalence can affect the positive predictive value of a test.

Treatment of an Abnormal Case

Evidence from clinical trials has given us drugs, treatments, therapies, devices and procedures that we could use to treat individual patients. Since epidemiology along cannot successfully define what is normal and what is abnormal; treatment of "clinically" abnormal cases need to be done using the treatment methods available.

Clinically, it may be meaningful to know that patients with hypertension need to be treated when blood pressure becomes equivalent or more than 140/90. Epidemiology along may not define with such narrow margin; clinical trials could provide best evidence of usefulness of a drug/s or treatment/s in lowering blood pressure and corresponding gain.

Likewise, diagnostic tests are also available to be able to diagnose clinically using microbiological, biochemical and other means so that one could successfully treat 'abnormal' or diseased cases.

Natural History of Disease

This deals with the latent period, pathological onset, presymptomatic stage → onset of signs and symptoms.

This also includes remissions and relapses.

Some diseases may regress spontaneously and some may progress aggressively and morality could occur.

Knowledge of disease is useful in its prevention for obvious reason. Epidemiological information could provide a sound ground for predicting prognosis and outcome of a given disease.

Epidemiological studies could help us know the natural history of disease.

This could mean that we will have to measure all possible clinical outcomes, e.g. complications and not just the morbidity and mortality associated with disease.

Nowadays, life table analysis have become available to predict the onset of events over time from the pattern of patients at risk. Therefore, in the follow-up of cohort of patients to determine prognosis bias can arise from the method of assembling the cohort and from incomplete follow-up.

How to Evaluate Effectiveness of Treatment?

No matter, how good the treatment is; and how high the efficacy of treatment is; its effectiveness may be low. This is determined by many factors including compliance.

Treatment used clinically, obviously, has to be effective. Effectiveness of a treatment refers to its ability to do well in real life situation. This signifies acceptance by the patients. Efficacy is measured in motivated, monitored and carefully selected patients.

Effectiveness measurement trials are sometimes also called pragmatic trials and these could be tagged with *pharmacovigilance* program. Adverse drug reactions can also be monitored along with effectiveness. Type of study designs exploring effectiveness are called *open label* studies. In such studies both investigators and participants know about what is being assigned what.

How to Prevent Disease in Clinical Practice?

Normally, principles of preventive medicines are described using the entire population and not the individual patients. Inside the hospitals, normally, the emphasis is on treatment and not on prevention.

That means, prevention is done at secondary or tertiary level.

However, even at clinical level many preventive strategies are being used now:
a. Newborns are screened for hypothyroidism.
b. Antenatal care in pregnancy and measuring their blood sugar to detect diabetes.
c. Screening eligible couples for *thalassemia* trait.

Emphasis is on identifying the "cases" and thus treat them. So this is obviously secondary level care. In tertiary care, focus is on treating cases to prevent complications.

Clinics as Centers of Preventive Medicine

a. Even health workers could advise people to quit smoking and studies have shown that even this may have good impact on their psyche. People may be motivated to quit smoking.

b. In memory clinics, apart from treatment of hypertension, diabetes and other risk factors leading to dementia; one could advise mathematics, puzzles and other games that could activate brain and help in preventing dementia.

How well is a subject classified into disease or non-disease group? "Ideally, all subjects who have the disease should be classified "having the disease" and vice versa practically, the ability to classify individuals into the correct disease status depends on the accuracy of the tests, among other things (Fig. 13.2).

Table 13.2: Examples of diagnostic tests

- Pap smear for cervical dysplasia or cervical cancer
- Fasting blood cholesterol for heart disease
- Fasting blood sugar for diabetes
- Blood pressure for hypertension
- Mammography for breast cancer
- PSA test for prostate cancer
- Fecal occult blood for colon cancer
- Ocular pressure for glaucoma
- PKU test for phenylketonuria in newborns
- TSH for hypothyroid and hyperthyroid

Relationship between Sensitivity and Specificity

There is a yin-yang relationship between sensitivity and specificity. Changing test cut-off values to increase the sensitivity will reduce the specificity, and vice versa. For example, the diabetes is diagnosed based on a fasting blood sugar ≥ 126 mg/dL. If we raise the cut-off to 180 mg/dL, we make it more difficult have a positive diabetes test, i.e. a diagnosis of DM.

We have made our test less sensitive (some true diabetics will not have blood sugar that high) and more specific (normal people may get their blood sugar to 126, but are unlikely to get it to 180). The opposite applies to lowering the cut-off: we become more sensitive but less specific. Sensitivity and specificity give us likelihood of the test result among persons known to be diseased or healthy. As clinicians, we need to know the opposite: the likelihood of being diseased or healthy among persons with a known test result. Consider: What is the likelihood that a person with a positive test will actually have the disease (i.e. what is the PV+) when the prevalence = 20% in a population of 10^4 .

Sensitivity = 90% and specificity = 90%

Bibliography

1. Beaglehole et al., Basic Epidemiology. World Health Organization, AITBS Publishers 2006 (Updated reprint), pp. 60–81.

2. Dhikav V. Basic and Clinical Epidemiology. AITBS Publishers New Delhi, India 2014, 1st edition, pp. 12–25.

3. https://onlinecourses.science.psu.edu/stat 509/node/148 (Downloaded on May 3rd 2017).

4. Prasad K. Evidence-based medicine in India. J Clin Epidemiol. 2013 Jan; 66(1):6-9. doi: 10.1016/j.j clinepi. 2012.07.006.

5. Schulzer M. Diagnostic tests: a statistical review. Muscle Nerve. 1994 Jul;17(7):815–819.

6. Screening and diagnostic tests. http://emedicine. medscape.com/article/773832-overview (Downloaded on May 3rd 2017).

7. Statistical methods for diagnostic agreements. http://www.john-uebersax.com/stat/agree. htm (Downloaded on May 3rd 2017).

Chapter 14

Surveys, Questionnaire and Scales

Learning objectives

Scales are commonly used tools in observational and analytical research. They could be comparative or non comparative. Selecting a scale or questionnaire depends upon the type of data, how much information is required and the statistical methods available. Scales could give valuable information about a topic and are common ways of doing observational research.

Survey

Broadly speaking, survey is a method of gathering data (can be qualitative or quantitative). Surveys present a set of questions to a subject who with his/her responses will provide data to a researcher. This method of doing research seems simple, but may have many possible pitfalls along the way. Data collection is done using standardized information questionnaires.

A questionnaire is appropriate when one wants information from a large number of people. It is done when someone has an understanding of the situation and can ask meaningful questions. Formulating a questionnaire can be challenging.

Why Develop Questionnaire?

When doing research; the information needed may be sensitive or private. People may be more willing to answer an anonymous questionnaire rather than personal one to one interviews. This may reduce bias.

Questionnaire help gathering data. Also they may translate opinions into action. They are hence very useful in making policy and improving the working conditions. In biomedical sciences, they can be very useful for screening or diagnostic purposes. Questionnaire can also be helpful in evaluation of health programs and measure of what they say they do. One would need to know how opinions and behaviors vary across different categories of people. This is especially true in social sciences or psychology/psychiatry.

Developing a Questionnaire

Questionnaire is developed to answer a question so that every potential respondent responds. The aim is to have a questionnaire that will interpreted in the same way, and responded accurately by all. Ideally all the participants should be willing to answer. Following are the useful tips while formulating a questionnaire:

a Avoid asking two questions at once (double-barreled question).

Example:
Do you feel that your skills in public speaking and leading new groups have increased as a result of new training?
Yes
No
Not sure
One can ask such a question

Ask each question separately:

a. Do you feel that your skills in public speaking have increased?
Yes
No
Not sure

b. Do you feel that your skills in leading new groups have increased?

Yes

No

Not sure

c. Do you feel, these changes are due to your training?

Yes

No

Not sure

While formulating questions; one should avoid jargon and technical language. For example, parents when they are coming to school after their child has passed 12th class is being counseled by the counselor:

Question

What kind of set experience would you prefer for your child?

Better Question

"What kind of Science, Engineering and Technology experience would you prefer for your child?"

One should always avoid imprecise questions

Imprecise: How would you describe your experience as a medical student?

Better: How would you describe your training experience while being at medical college Rohtak, Haryana?

It is important to know that while asking the questions, the more specific you are about what you want to know, the more useful the answer will be. Also, one should avoid vague or ambiguous words and concepts.

Vague: How many times did you eat together as a family last week?

Better: How many meals did you eat together as a family at home last week?

More specific: How many meals did you sit down to eat at home as a family last week?

One should avoid specificity that limits the potential for reliable recall. Example is given below:

Too specific: How may hours did you contribute to community service last year?

This question is also ambiguous since "community service" is not defined and may mean different things to different people. One can include dates to specify anytime frame, in 2015; January–June 2016, etc.

Basic Instruments of Surveys and Structured Interviews

Not only framing of the question is important in surveys and structured interviews response, i.e. wording the answer is important as well. Wording the response is as important as clear wording in the question. Make the answer options clear, logical, comparable and mutually exclusive. Also one should include both positive and negative sides in the question stem and all possible answer options.

Poor

Do you agree that your friends club needs to meet once per month?

• Agree

• Disagree

Better

Do you agree or disagree that our friends club needs to meet once per month?

• Agree

• Disagree

• No opinion

Another option: How often do you think our friends club should meet?

• More than once a month

• Once a month

• Less than once a month

Such questions are appropriate when one wants to collects information from many people same time. Also when one has some understanding of the situation and can ask meaningful questions. This works when the information is sensitive or private and people may be more willing to answer an anonymous questionnaire; may reduce bias. To do this, there are many types of surveys (Table 14.1).

Table 14.1: Types of surveys

- Self-administered surveys
- Face-to-face interviews
- Telephone surveys
- Computer assisted and web-based
- E-mail surveys

One should determine if the focus is on any survey or questionnaire. It is crucial to know how to ask the questions in written and spoken form. The way you ask the questions determines the answers. One should identify the questionnaire's specific purpose/s. Be sure to have the specific objectives of the questionnaire. One should thoroughly know the respondents and standardize the interviewer.

Before starting the actual study, one has to standardize the response format as well. One should ask questions in a social, cultural, and economic context depending upon the theme of the questionnaire. It may be totally medically/health oriented too. During the study, one has to keep confidentiality of the participants. A signed consent is a must before taking interviews.

In the beginning when the study has not been started one should not forget to include a letter of introduction or presentation about the study. Open questions may yield more information but are difficult to codify, enter, and analyze. Closed questions are less informative but easy to codify, enter, and analyze (Tables 14.2 and 14.3).

Self-Administered Questionnaires

Self-administered questionnaire is a format in which the respondents complete on their own. It is best designed for measuring variables with numerous values or response categories. Also, these are good for describing characteristics

Table 14.2: Advantages and disadvantages of questionnaire

Inaccurate/dishonest	Inaccurate/dishonest responses
Easy to analyze responses	Chance of none of the choices being appropriate
Stimulates recall	Biases response to what you're looking for Misses unintended outcomes
Provides anonymity	Wording of the questionnaire can bias the respondent
Relatively inexpensive	Low response rate
Easy to analyze and interpret	Mistakes in filling up questionnaire

Table 14.3: Advantages and disadvantages of open and closed ended questions

Can get unintended or unanticipated results	More difficult to answer
Wide variety of answers	May be harder to categorize for interpretation
Answers in participants' "voices"	More difficult for people who don't write much

of a large population. Studying 'private' or 'difficult' behaviors could best be done by them. We need to know that the response rates tend to be lowest for mailed questionnaires. The response rate could be as low as 20–30% and the low response rate affects generalizability.

Closed-ended items could limit the researcher's ability to generalize the findings of research. One may have to adjust for differences in respondents, clarify the misunderstood items and also, explain the ambiguity. Hence, it may not be suitable for all audiences.

Computer Questionnaire

Computer questionnaire is a way to create and administer self-administered questionnaires. This is a common tool for marketing researchers find response rates increase. The questionnaires (especially short ones) can be sent via email or one can provide internet link to site which hosts survey.

Web-Based Survey

Web-based survey can be created at free websites nowadays or alternatively one can hire a commercial company (www. hostedsurvey.com) to get the questionnaire made. They allow for instant data coding. One would need to be able to write code or use software. It may be less time consuming and costs may be nominal. However, the access could be an issue and this can affect generalizability. Variation in computer ownership and usage or internet access can affect responses. Also the reading of questionnaire items in a face-to-face or telephone situation could yield different responses.

Unstructured or in-depth Interview

Unstructured or in-depth interview is suited for exploratory research. This could be done either with one person or in focus groups. One should include open-ended items as it is difficult to standardize. It is good for complex situations.

Structured Interview

This involves considering the role of interviewer as the style and personal characteristics of each interviewer differs. It is also influenced by the process. Hence, the training is critical. One has to follow the wording and record the responses. General Social Survey could be an example of such a survey. Response rates tend to be highest with face-to-face interviews. However, it is time consuming and yield is smaller.

Telephonic Surveys

Telephonic surveys are most popular and are less costly, less time consuming, less subjective to interviewer bias as compared to face-to-face and are often conducted with the help of computers nowadays. Telephonic surveys can probe for information/clarification and the threshold time is about 20 minutes.

Making a Questionnaire

Making a questionnaire could be challenging but regardless of survey type, construct in a way that allows for candid answers accurately and consistently. Also, the questionnaire must address goals, hypotheses, research questions, etc.

While formulating, one should list the set of research questions, hypotheses and consider how others have measured the same. At least one questionnaire item for each variable should be there. Also, one should operationalize the concept and outline what one wishes to cover. Attitudes, feelings, opinions and behaviors should be taken into account. Demographics should be noted.

Designing a Questionnaire

Demographic details, such as age, income, education, political beliefs, and sexual orientation are important. The following must be kept in mind:

a. Beginning of each section, should have clear instructions as to how to use the questionnaire.

b. Length of questionnaire should be an issue (i.e. it should not be too lengthy). Time to construct and time for respondents to complete should be pretested.

c. Font, spacing, format and the vocabulary and grammar to the population be surveyed should be kept in mind.

d. For studies within a specific organization, one should use the vocabulary/jargon used in that organization. Also one should be careful to avoid language that is familiar to one, but might not be to others. Avoid unnecessary abbreviations.

e. One should avoid ambiguity, confusion, and vagueness *in the questionnaire and* make sure it is absolutely clear what you are asking and how you want it answered. Avoid indefinite words or response categories.

f. One should avoid double-barreled questions and make each question about one and only one topic. It is important to know that the respondent is an expert on themselves.

g. Avoid asking questions beyond a respondent's capabilities. Naturally, people have cognitive limitations, especially when it comes to memory and other skills.

h. While asking questions, false information should be avoided. Also, one should avoid asking negatives and especially double negatives.

Construction of the questionnaire is the key to valid and reliable research. It should be well written and should have manageable questions.

Issues

The key to a successful questionnaire is that one should be getting the clear response. Limiting the response, too much of length, too intrusive and personal questions and private thoughts could be counter-productive.

Qualities of a Questionnaire

The questionnaire should be able to ask the purposeful questions. The questions should be concrete. The following are the additional features:

- Time periods
- Conventional language
- Complete sentences
- Avoid abbreviations
- Review questions with experts/potential respondents
- Shorter questions
- Avoid two-edged/negative questions
- Adopt/adapt questions used successfully in other questionnaires.

One should specify the information that needs to be sought. Also one needs to determine the type of questionnaire and method of administration. The content of individual questions should be finalized and pretested too. One will have to determine the form of response to each question and the wording of each question should be such that as to suit the potential respondents.

Rating Scales

One will have to include a label for each scale category and keep the order of the scale same throughout the questionnaire. It could be kept in mind that the odd number of options allows people to select a middle option and the even number may force respondents to take sides. The number of points on the scale depends upon the amount of differentiation (Three, four, or five categories are common).

It is very important to balance the scale with an equal number of positive and negative options. "No opinion" or "uncertain" are not part of a scale. They are placed off to the side or in a separate column. All choices should refer to the same thing/concept.

Poor

If one has to rate in overall, how would rate your experience of youth icons of India?

- Excellent
- Very good
- Good
- Fair
- Poor.

Better

Overall, how would you rate your experience of youth icons of India?

- Very good
- Good
- Fair
- Poor
- Very poor.

Make sure the response scale matches the question.

Poor

To what extent do you think the workshop on biostatistics helped you develop your leadership skills?

- Excellent
- Very good
- Good
- Fair
- Poor.

Better

To what extent do you think the workshop on biostatistics helped you develop your leadership skills?

- Very great extent
- Great extent
- Some extent

- Little extent
- Very little extent.

Pilot Testing

Always pretest the proforma and it should be discussed with people who are in know-how of the subject. Once the content is finalized it should be pretested in the participants. One of the major aims is to know if the participants understood the questions or not. Also, do the meaning of question appear same to all the participants or not. How long does it take to fill the proforma should be known.

Bibliography

1. Developing a questionnaire. http://libweb. surrey.ac.uk/library/skills/Introduction% 20to%20 Research%20and%20 Managing% 20Information%20Leicester/page_49.htm (Accessed online on February 1st 2017).

2. How to Develop a Questionnaire for Research http://www.wikihow.com/Develop-a-Questionnaire-for-Research (Accessed online on February 1st 2017).

3. Questionnaire design. http://www.fao.org/ docrep/w3241e/w3241e05.htm (Accessed online on February 1st 2017).

Validating in Medical Research

Learning objectives

Validity is, in general, an indicator of sound is the scientific research. It deals with both the design and methods of research. If the research is valid, then findings represent the phenomena one is measuring.

Reliability *on the other hand,* refers to *consistency* and *repeatability*. A reliable assessment provides a consistent picture of what students know, understand, and are able to do. An assessment that is highly reliable is not necessarily valid. However, for an assessment to be valid, it must also be reliable.

INTRODUCTION

These two terms, **reliability** and **validity**, are often used interchangeably when they are not related to statistics. When critical readers of statistics use these terms, however, they refer to different properties of the statistical or experimental method.

Last defines validity as the degree to which a measurement measures what it purports to measure. For example, if a weighing machine measures the weight of lean teen age girl as 120 kg, it is not valid. Similarly, if the same machine gives reading as 60 kg, 70 kg, 75 kg and 90 kg on 4 other separate measurements; it would be evident that this is neither reliable nor valid. So, it can be termed *the degree to which the data measure what they were intended to measure*. It means in other words, the results of a measurement correspond to the true state of the phenomenon being measured. This is also commonly known as 'accuracy'. It denotes the extent to which an instrument is measuring what it is supposed to measure (Fig. 15.1).

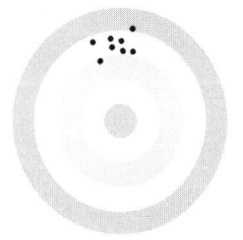 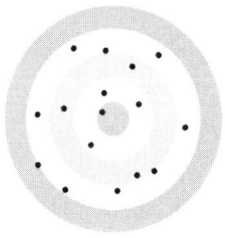 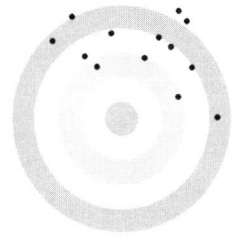 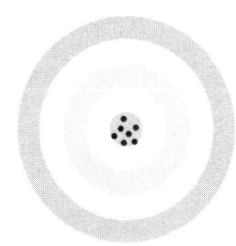

| Reliable not valid | Not reliable but valid | Not reliable and not valid | Reliable and valid |
| precise not accurate | not precise but accurate | not precise and not accurate | precise and accurate |

Fig. 15.1: For the measurements to be acceptable, they should be valid and reliable. Validity means, the extent to which the measurements can measure what they are supposed to measure. For example, if the blood pressure of a patient is 140/90, and the machine gives a reading of 120/80; naturally it is not valid instrument. Similarly, upon repeated measurements, the instruments should provide the similar readings. For example, the readings taken by blood pressure instrument of a patient with hypertension (blood pressure = 180/100 mm Hg) should be same regardless of the number of times they are taken

Evaluating Validity and Reliability

Evaluating the validity and reliability of the scientific information is a crucial step in evidence-based medical practice. *Bias* is any deviation of results or inferences from the truth because of the way/s in which the study is conducted.

It is important to remember that bias does not necessarily carry an allegation of prejudice as is often assumed, e.g. investigators' desire for particular results, etc. but it can be as a result of several issues.

While going through the published literature; the job of the critical readers is to determine whether the weakness is serious enough to warrant reinterpretation of the study's finding or not. We need to question whether the study measures what it intended to measure and whether the researchers have accounted for the bias and confounding variables or not.

Internal vs External Validity

Validity is of two main types: internal and external (Fig. 15.2). Internal validity is the experimenter measuring the effect of the independent variable on the dependent variable?

So, the internal validity deals with "keeping the house in order", i.e. whether the methods and materials used in research have been

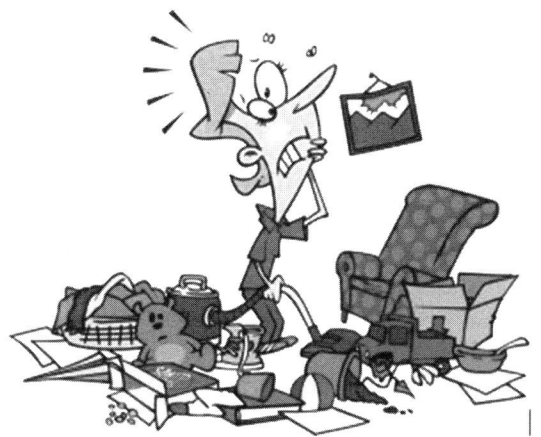

Fig. 15.2: Keeping house in order reflects good internal validity during research. Proper sampling, organizing data, looking for bias and good study designs can enhance internal validity

properly standardized or not. If the results of the study can be generalized to the population, then this is known as external validity.

Clinical Significance

After assessing the internal and external validity of a research article, the next step is to determine whether the research is clinically significant or not. One should determine if the results of the research are applicable to patient setting or the clinical scenario. Whatever be the outcome of the research, one can ask if the experimental treatment or the test would be available in clinic/hospital? If so, will it be cost effective? The answers to these questions are largely individual as practitioners have varying thresholds of acceptable risk and cost restraints when applying a new treatment or using a new diagnostic tool. Please note that clinical significance is different from statistical significance.

Validity in the era of Evidence-Based Medicine

Validity refers to the accuracy of inferences drawn from an assessment. It is the degree to which the assessment measures what it is intended to measure. The validity is about providing strong evidence for research and practice. Naturally, evidence-centered research design boosts validity.

Reliability should be differentiated from validity. Reliability is the extent to which the variables are free from random error, usually determined by measuring the variables more than once.

Systematic Error

Systematic error has the sources of error including the style of measurement, tendency. This creeps into the system and then whole measurements could become faulty.

Systematic error is constant throughout a set of readings. This may result from the equipment which is incorrectly calibrated or how measurements are performed, e.g. a blood pressure instrument that gives wrong readings. This causes the mean of measured values to depart from correct value. One would have to keep a high index of suspicion as it may be difficult to spot presence of systematic errors in an experiment.

Examining Internal Validity

As stated, there are two types of validity: internal validity and external validity. *The internal validity must be established before external validity.* Internal validity tries to determine the connection between the independent variable and dependent variable in the experimental set-up. This is very important in medicine when the investigator tries to ask a question "Did the treatment cause the effect?" One can use the questions below to help determine internal validity. Questions that examine internal validity:

a. *Research question*: This is the first step in medical research where one tends to define the research question first. So one should ask: is there a clear research question? If no, this is a big threat to internal validity.

b. *Question-method mismatch*: Does the research method match the question? If no, then it can be a troublesome research.

c. *Control group*: This is one of the most important step. Absence of control group can land any researcher in medicine in trouble. So one should ask oneself if there was any control group? If no, then comparison is difficult.

d. *Representativeness*: One should ask if the sample is drawn from the population to which the researchers seek to generalize the results? if no? then this can be particularly problematic because if internal validity is not there but external validity will definitely be poor.

e. *Randomization and statistical analysis*: Have randomization and/or blinding employed when appropriate? How is the analysis performed, and what statistical methods are used? In treatment studies, are all participants accounted for and analyzed according to intention to treat? One should ensure if the conclusions are supported by the study's findings?

External

External validity is nothing but the extent to which the results be generalized to the wider population? While checking the validity, several things need to be taken into account:

a. *Criterion Validity*

This is a method for assessing the validity of an instrument by comparing its scores with another criterion known already to be a measure of the same trait or skill. Criterion-related validity is usually expressed as a correlation between the test in question and the criterion that we wish to measure.

b. *Concurrent Validity*

The extent to which a procedure correlates with the current behavior of subjects. This can also project the extent to which a procedure allows accurate predictions about a subject's future behavior.

c. *Content Validity*

Whether the individual items of a test represent what you actually want to assess or not.

d. *Construct Validity*

The extent to which a test measures a theoretical construct or attribute is called construct validity. It is important to know that some abstract concepts, such as intelligence, self-concept, motivation, aggression and creativity that can be measured by some types of psychological instruments in practice. So, the construct validity will be said to exist if the said test measures the said concept. A test's construct validity is often assessed by its convergent and discriminant validity.

Factors Affecting Validity

1. Test-related factors
2. The criterion to which you compare your instrument may not be well enough established
3. Intervening events
4. Reliability

Bibliography

1. Concept of validity. http://www.statsdirect. com/help/basics/validity.htm (Downloaded on May 3rd 2017).

2. Measuring validity. https://explorable.com/ statistical-validity (Downloaded on May 3rd 2017).

3. Statistical methods: validity and reliability. http://onlinelibrary.wiley.com/doi/10.1111/ j.1553-2712.1997.tb03723.x/pdf (Downloaded on May 3rd 2017).

4. Validity and reliability explained. https://allpsych. com/researchmethods/validityreliability/ (Downloaded on May 3rd 2017).

5. Validity and reliability. http://web.cortland. edu/ andersmd/STATS/valid.html (Downloaded on May 3rd 2017).

6. Validity. http://www.statisticssolutions. com/ validity/(Downloaded on May 3rd 2017).

Testing Reliability in Medical Research

Learning objectives

Reliability refers to the extent to which a scale produces consistent results in the measurements of intended variables, if the measurements are repeated a number of times. The analysis on reliability is called reliability analysis. Reliability analysis is determined by obtaining the proportion of systematic variation in a scale, which can be done by determining the association between the scores obtained from different administrations of the scale. Thus, if the association in reliability analysis is high, the scale yields consistent results and is therefore reliable.

What is Reliability?

Reliability is also known as 'reproducibility' or 'precision'. In other words, the reliability is the consistency of measurements (Fig. 16.1).

A reliable test produces similar scores across various conditions and situations, including different evaluators and testing environments. Commonly used terms while describing conversations or objects are *"She has a valid point"* or *"My new laptop is unreliable as it is a good brand"*.

In science, one often refers the validity and reliability as: *"The conclusion of the study was not valid"* or *"the findings of the study were not reliable"*.

In broader terms the reliability refers to the consistency of a research study or measuring test. For example, if a person weighs themselves during the course of a day they would expect to see a similar reading. Scales which measured weight differently each time would be of little use. The same analogy could be applied to a tape measure which measures inches differently each time it was used. It would not be considered reliable.

Correlation Coefficient as an Indicator of Reliability

If findings from research are replicated consistently they are reliable. A correlation coefficient can be used to assess the degree of reliability. If a test is reliable it should show a high positive correlation. Of course, it is unlikely the exact same results will be obtained each time as participants and situations vary, but a strong positive correlation between the results of the same test indicates reliability (Fig. 16.2).

Errors

An error is the amount by which a taken observation differs from the expected value. Naturally, the later observation

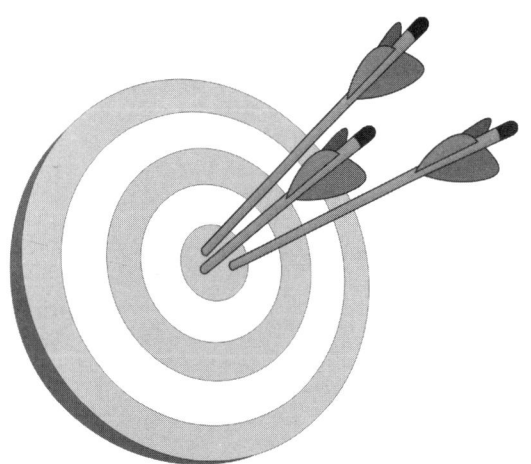

Fig. 16.1: For a measurement to be valid and reliable, it should be able to hit the "bull's eye" always

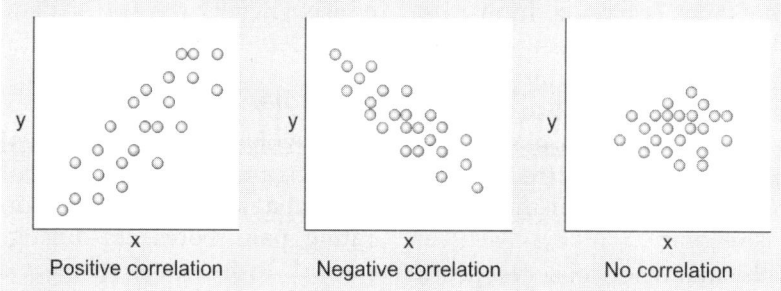

Fig. 16.2: A high positive correlation indicates a high degree of reliability

pertains to the whole population. If the sample has been chosen properly the sample mean could act as a good estimator of the population mean.

Random error is called the chance fluctuations. They tend to cancel out over repeated measurements.

The systematic error represents the fluctuations that are slanted in a particular direction. This is also known as "bias".

Why do Reliability Testing?

Validity and reliability are needed for hypothesis testing, i.e. without validity and reliability one cannot test an hypothesis. Moreover, without hypothesis testing, one cannot support a theory. Without a supported theory one cannot explain why events occur. Additionally, without adequate explanation one cannot develop effective technologies.

From an experimental standpoint, reliability is the degree of stability expected when a measurement is repeated under identical conditions. In other words, it is the degree to which the results obtained from a measurement procedure can be replicated.

For example, if blood pressure of 1 elderly patient is measured by 5 different doctors, then naturally different doctors have used the same instruments so you expect the reading to vary. But it may not be the case if the instrument is reliable!

So reliability is the extent to which repeated measurements of a stable phenomenon by different people and instruments, at different times and places get similar results.

Types of Reliabilities

There are two types of reliability like validity (internal and external reliability). Internal reliability assesses the consistency of results across items within a test. The external reliability refers to the extent to which a measure varies from one use to another.

Test retest measures the stability of the test overtime. Inter-rater reliability can be an estimate of the degree to which different raters agree on the same estimate.

Test-retest Reliability

Test-retest reliability suggests that subjects tend to obtain the same score when tested at different times. In other words, this represents the extent to which the scores on the same variable correlate with each other on two different measurements at two different times.

In practical terms, the respondents are administered identical sets of a scale of items at two different times under equivalent conditions.

The degree of similarity between the two measurements is determined by computing a correlation coefficient; the higher the correlation coefficient in reliability analysis, the greater the reliability.

It should be kept in mind that the rest-retest reliability is sensitive to the time interval between testing. The initial measurement may alter the characteristic being measured in test-retest reliability in reliability analysis.

The test-retest method assesses the external consistency of a test. This refers to the degree to which different raters give consistent estimates of the same behavior. Inter-rater reliability can be used for interviews.

Note, it can also be called inter-observer reliability when referring to observational research. Here researcher when observe the same behavior independently (to avoided bias) and compare their data. If the data is similar then it is reliable.

It is noteworthy that where observer scores do not significantly correlate then reliability can be improved by training the observers in the observation techniques being used and making sure everyone agrees with them.

Split Half Reliability (Internal Consistency)

This is also sometimes referred to as *internal consistency*. This indicates that subjects' scores on some trials consistently match their scores on other trials. This measures the extent to which all the parts of the test contribute equally to what is being measured. It is a measure of internal reliability.

In split half test, assignments of subjects are assumed random. The observations should be independent of each other. The variances should be equivalently assumed.

Thus internal consistency measures the extent to which the scores on the items correlate with each other and thus all measure the true score rather than reflecting random error. Internal consistency is measured as Chronbach alpha (coefficient alpha).

Practically, the items on the scale are divided into two halves and the resulting half scores are correlated in reliability analysis. High correlations between the halves indicate high internal consistency in reliability analysis. The scale items can be split into halves, based on odd and even numbered items in reliability analysis. The limitation in this analysis is that the outcomes will depend on how the items are split. In order to overcome this limitation, coefficient alpha or *Cronbach's alpha* is used in reliability analysis.

In reliability analysis, internal consistency is used to measure the reliability of a summated scale where several items are summed to form a total score. This measure of reliability in reliability analysis focuses on the internal consistency of the set of items forming the scale.

Inter-rater Reliability

This involves having two raters independently observe and record observations, e.g. clinical dementia rating, medial temporal lobe atrophy rating, pain scores, etc. during the same time period. In practical terms it deals with the extent the scores counted by coders correlate with each other. It is expressed as Cohen's kappa.

Since it deals with the raters it is also called inter-rater agreement. Inter-rater reliability helps to understand whether or not two or more raters or interviewers administrate the same form to the same people homogeneously. This is done in order to establish the extent of consensus that the instrument has been used by those who administer it.

This is based upon certain assumptions like the errors should be uncorrelated. Also the coding done should have the same meaning across items.

Alternate form Reliability

Alternate form reliability is also known as equivalent forms reliability or parallel forms reliability. This is obtained by administering two equivalent tests to the same group of examinees. Items are matched for difficulty on each test. It is necessary that the time frame between giving the two forms be as short as possible. The score one gets when one does administers a test consists of two parts: the true score and the error score. This form of reliability gives the margin of error that one could expect in an individual test score because of imperfect reliability of the test.

Bibliography

1. Precision of measurement. http://www.sportsci.org/resource/stats/precision.html (Accessed online dated February 7th 2017).
2. Reliability analysis. http://www.statisticssolutions.com/directory-of-statistical-analyses-reliability-analysis/(Accessed online dated February 7th 2017).
3. Statistical reliability. https://explorable.com/statistical-reliability (Accessed online dated February 7th 2017).

17

Data Collection

Learning objectives

Data can be collected by various methods, e.g. experiments, interviews, questionnaires (especially in neurology, psychiatry and psychology) and surveys (in social sciences), etc. Observations, focus Groups and Case Studies are other methods of collecting data. The data can be primary or secondary; each one has its pros and cons but the first type is preferable. Also, the collected data can be qualitative or quantitative.

Data

Goal of research is to draw conclusions. It starts with the question: What did the study mean? What, if any, is the cause and effect of the outcome?

The data can be:

Quantitative: These include numbers, tests, counting, etc. For example, blood pressure, blood sugar, liver and kidney function test values, etc.

Qualitative: These include words, images, observations, conversations, photographs, etc.

Data Variables

Independent variable: The variable in the study under consideration. Independent variables are the cause for the outcome for the study.

Dependent variable: The variable being affected by the independent variable. The effect of the study depends upon these variables, e.g. vitamin D status.

As a general rule; the data should not be contaminated by poor measurement or errors in procedure. Also one should eliminate confounding variables from study or minimize effects on variables. The sample selected should have representativeness. For example, does it represent the population one is studying? To be able to get results one would want, random sampling techniques are the best as they minimize the bias.

Types of Data

Data can be primary or secondary. The primary data is collected by the investigator but the secondary data is collected by someone and is analyzed and interpreted by someone else. Obviously, it is less hectic to work on the secondary data but it has its pros and cons.

Primary Data

- Surveys
- Focus groups
- Questionnaires
- Personal interviews
- Experiments and observational study.

Secondary Data

- County health departments
- Vital statistics—birth, death certificates
- Hospital, clinic, school nurse records
- Private and foundation databases
- City and county governments
- Surveillance data from state government programs
- Federal agency statistics—Census, NIH, etc.

Limitations of Primary Data

Primary data is the best possible data as it is collected by the investigator. Naturally it depends upon the time and money for the research. The main advantage is that one would be designing own collection instrument and selecting population/sample. This will have to be preceded by pretesting/piloting the instrument to workout sources of bias etc. This may need loads of money, resources and time.

Advantages of Secondary Data

The main advantage of using the secondary data is that one would not need to reinvent the wheel. That means, one can use something that had already been done. It will save time and money in simple terms. In practical terms if one is using the secondary data for conducting some research; even if one would have to pay for the data access, it is cheaper in terms of money than collecting one's own data. Primary data collection is very time consuming. It is important to know that one should not always try and find faults with primary data; it may be very accurate too. This is specially the case when a government agency has collected the data, then lot of time and money has gone into it. Secondary data may have good exploratory value as exploring research questions and formulating hypothesis to test could become much easier.

Drawbacks of Secondary Data

Important questions such as when was it collected and for how long are not clear. It may even be out of date for what one would want to analyze! Importantly, it may not have been collected long enough for detecting trends. One of the major worry is that if the data set was complete or not. There may be missing information on some observations. Unless such missing information is caught and corrected for, analysis will be biased. Also one would have to find out confounding problems, e.g. sample selection bias, source choice bias, etc. One would have to find especially in a time series, if observations dropout overtime or not. Also the consistency and reliability could be an issue. One would have to ensure if the study subjects dropped out overtime and if there were other variations important too.

Self-Reported Data

Self-reported data is unstructured or semi-unstructured as it is based upon self-report techniques, e.g. interviews or verbal communication between research and subject; commonly used in exploratory and descriptive studies.

Self-report data can be gathered either by oral interview or by written questionnaire. The self-report method is strong with respect to its directness and flexibility if we want to know what people think, feel, or believe (qualitative data) the most direct means of gathering the information is to ask them about it.

Unstructured Interview

This is subject's world view; open-ended questions with probes and prompting are provided. This is qualitative and is often recorded as an audiotape.

Semi-structured Interview

This is also one subject's list of topics or questions for discussion with additional probes, also known as topic guide; uses both open and close-ended questions. It is also taped.

Structured Interview

This is also one subject's view; specific questions asked in consistent order using the same words each time; no variation from questions and no explanation of unclear questions.

Focus Group Interview

This involves 5 to 15 subjects in a group and the interviewer/moderator asks open-ended questions; efficient yet some individuals inhibited by others in the group.

Disadvantages

Self-reported data shares a number of weaknesses. The most serious issue is the question of the validity and accuracy of self-report. How can we really be sure that respondents feel or act the way they say they do? Also how can the information that respondents provide, particularly if the questions could potentially require them to reveal an unpopular position on a controversial issues could be trusted?

Sampling

Sampling is the task of accurately acquiring the necessary data in order to form a representative view of the problem. This is much more difficult to do than is generally realized. To be able to sample the population effectively, one should:

- State the objectives of the survey
- Define the target population
- Define the data to be collected
- Define the variables to be determined
- Define the required precision and accuracy
- Define the measurement 'instrument'
- Define the sample size and sampling method, then select the sample.

Data Distributions

When one samples from a population, one can show it by a plotted distribution known as a histogram. A histogram is the distribution of frequency of occurrence of a certain variable within a specified range.

Statistics is a tool for converting *data* into *information*: But where then does *data* come from? How is it gathered? How do we ensure its accurate? Is the data reliable? Is it representative of the population from which it was drawn? This chapter explores some of these issues.

Data Collection

Data collection means gathering information to address those critical questions that one has identified earlier in the research process. It has to be a systematic and ordered process. Noting down details on piece of paper can be confusing and misleading.

Data Collection Plan

To plan data collection, one must think about the questions to be answered and the information sources available. Then one should begin to think ahead about how the information could be organized, analyzed, interpreted and then reported to various audiences.

Data Collection Methods

There are many methods available to gather information, and a wide variety of information sources. One has to keep several things in mind:

1. Clearly define the goals and objectives of the data collection. This is best done using a standardized proforma.
2. Reach understanding and agreement on operational definitions and methodology for the data collection plan. In the absence of such definition, things could easily get cluttered.
3. Ensure the collected data or measurements have repeatability, reproducibility, accuracy, and stability.

Value of Data

The information one has collected is the evidence one will have available to answer the evaluation questions. This is stored for the long time even after the research is over. It is important to know that the poor evidence is information which cannot be trusted. This information can be limited, or simply is not relevant to the questions asked. Good evidence is information that comes from reliable sources. Thoroughness in data collection and the use of standardized methods that address important questions enhances value of data.

There are many methods used to collect or obtain data for statistical analysis. Three of the most popular methods are:

1. Direct observation
2. Experiments
3. Surveys.

A *survey* solicits information from people, e.g. Gallup polls; pre-election polls; marketing surveys. The response rate (i.e. the proportion of all people selected who complete the survey) is a key survey parameter.

Surveys may be administered in a variety of ways, e.g.
- Personal interview,
- Telephone interview,
- Self-administered questionnaire, and
- Internet.

Questionnaire

This is a very popular method of eliciting response in the medical research. This may be a qualitative method but it is often rewarding. Key design principles:
- Keep the questionnaire as short as possible.
- Ask short, simple, and clearly worded questions.
- Start with demographic questions to help respondents get started comfortably.
- Use dichotomous (yes|no) and multiple choice questions.
- Use open-ended questions cautiously.
- Avoid using leading-questions.
- Pretest a questionnaire on a small number of people.
- Think about the way you intend to use the collected data when preparing the questionnaire.

A questionnaire is done in group or individuals and is usually easy with group. Personal contact with subjects is achieved and the responses can be obtained by mail as well. We should have a response rate of at least 60% to avoid response bias. If we were to send the questionnaire, a cover letter stating completion and return of questionnaire should be sent. Consent of subject is a must and he/she can drop off and pick-up in person or e-mail. Postcards were popular in the past. Their advantages include they are cheaper, anonymity, no interviewer bias, etc.

Good Data Collection

A good data collection plan is free from bias, and confounding. It should have control of extraneous variables. The data collection should be aimed to achieve statistical precision as to test the stated hypothesis. It is important to understand *bias* which occurs observations favor some individuals in the population over

others. *Confounding* occurs when the effects of two or more variables cannot be separated. An *extraneous variables* is any variable that has an effect on the dependent variable. One would need to identify and minimize these variables. Remember "Precise" means sharply defined or measured. "Accurate" means truthful or correct.

Developing a Data Collection Plan

One would have to identify types of data needed for the study to begin. Also one would have to select the types of measures to measure each variable would be described in. Selection or the development of instrument will be next goal. It is important to know that one would have to secure written permission to use each instrument. Pilot testing of the researcher-developed instrument and revised plan will be needed. Next comes the development of data collection forms and procedures. Surely, it will have to be implemented.

Talk to the Data

Talking to the data means identifying the data which has been used to describe characteristics of sample (e.g. demographics—age, gender, education background, marital status, etc.) and subsequently testing hypothesis or answering research questions. Control for extraneous variables is a must and one must measure as many as possible. One the data has been talked to, it is turn to analyze and interpret the same.

Pilot Testing

One would have to pretest and revise plan/instrument based on theoretical framework of study. Pilot test is done on small scale and measurements are evaluated before administration in large group.

Errors in Data Acquisition

Errors arise from the recording of incorrect responses, due to incorrect measurements being taken because of faulty equipment, mistakes made during transcription from primary sources, inaccurate recording of data due to misinterpretation of terms, or inaccurate responses to questions concerning sensitive issues. Two major types of error can arise when a sample of observations is taken from a population: *sampling error* and *nonsampling error*.

Sampling error refers to differences between the sample and the population that exist only because of the observations that happened to be selected for the sample. Random and we have no control over.

Nonsampling errors are more serious and are due to mistakes made in the acquisition of data or due to the sample observations being selected improperly. Most likely caused be poor planning, sloppy work, etc.

Bibliography

1. Glesne C, Peshkin A. Becoming qualitative researchers: An introduction. White Plains, NY: Longman Publishing (1992).

2. Morse JM. Critical issues in qualitative research methods. Thousand Oaks, CA: Sage Publications (1993).

3. Patton MQ. Qualitative evaluation and research methods (2nd ed.). Thousand Oaks, CA: Sage Publications (1990).

4. Rubin HJ, Rubin IS. Qualitative interviewing. Thousand, Oaks, CA: Sage Publications (1995).

Clinical Epidemiology
Tools in Medical Research

Learning objectives

Epi—means "on, upon, befall" and demo—means "people, population, man" logy—means study of. So this is the science of demographics. Some see epidemiology as science; others see it as a method. Generally epidemiology is seen as a scientific method to investigate disease

Epidemiologists are not concerned with an individual's disease as clinicians do, but with a population' distribution of the disease and its determinants in person, place, and time.

History of Epidemiology

The Greek physician Hippocrates is sometimes said to be the father of Epidemiology. He is the first person known to have examined the relationships between the occurrence of disease and environmental influences. He coined the terms *endemic* (for diseases usually found in some places but not in others) and *epidemic* (for disease that are seen at some times but not others).

One of the earliest theories on the origin of disease was that it was primarily the fault of human luxury. This was expressed by philosophers, such as Plato and Rousseau, and social critics like Jonathan Swift.

In the medieval Islamic world, physicians discovered the contagious nature of infectious disease. In particular, the Persian physician Avicenna, considered a "father of modern medicine," in *The Canon of Medicine* (1020s), discovered the contagious nature of tuberculosis and sexually transmitted disease, and the distribution of disease through water and soil.

Avicenna stated that bodily secretion is contaminated by foul foreign earthly bodies before being infected. He introduced the method of quarantine as a means of limiting the spread of contagious disease.

He also used the method of risk factor analysis, and proposed the idea of a syndrome in the diagnosis of specific diseases.

History of Clinical Epidemiology

Dr. John Snow is famous for his investigations into the causes of the 19th Century Cholera epidemics. He began with a comparison between the death rates from areas supplied by two adjacent water companies in Southwark.

His identification of the Broad Street pump as the cause of the SoHo epidemic is considered the classic example of epidemiology. He used chlorine in an attempt to clean the water and had the handle removed, thus ending the outbreak. This has been perceived as a major event in the history of public health and can be regarded as the founding event of the science of epidemiology.

Epidemiology, broadly spoken is an investigative method used to detect the cause or source of diseases, disorders, syndromes, conditions, or perils that cause pain, injury illness, disability, or death in human populations or groups.

Epidemiology is study of the nature, cause, control, and determinants of the frequency and distribution of disease, disability, and death in human populations. Epidemiology involves characterizing the distribution of heath status, diseases, or other health problems in terms of age, sex, race, geography, religion, education, occupation, behaviors, time, place, person, etc. This characterization is done in order to explain the distribution of a disease or health related problems in terms of the causal factors. Epidemiology serves as the foundation and logic of interventions made in the interest of public health and preventive medicine.

It is considered a cornerstone methodology of public health research, and is highly regarded in evidence-based medicine for identifying risk factors for disease and determining optimal treatment approaches to clinical practice.

In the work of communicable and non-communicable diseases, the work of epidemiologists range from outbreak investigation to study design, data collection and analysis including the development of statistical models to test hypotheses and the documentation of results for submission to peer-reviewed journals.

Epidemiologists may draw on a number of other scientific disciplines, such as biology in understanding disease processes and social science disciplines including sociology and philosophy in order to better understand proximate and distal risk factors.

Why Epidemiology?

Epidemiology as a science is needed to explain the etiology (cause) of a single disease or group of diseases using information management. It is valuable to determine if data are consistent with proposed hypothesis. To provide a basis for developing control measures and prevention procedures for groups and at risk populations.

Epidemiological interpretations are based upon some assumptions, e.g. assumption include disease does not occur randomly and the disease has identifiable causes which can be altered and therefore prevent disease from developing. Health-related states or events: health status, diseases, death, other implications of disease such as disability, residual dysfunction, complication, recurrence, but also causes of death, behavior, provision and use of health services.

Types of Epidemiology

Descriptive epidemiology deals with the health status of a population, and works to assess the public health importance of diseases. So the descriptive epidemiology describes the occurrence of disease (cross-sectional). It also deals with the natural history of disease. Analytic epidemiology on the other hand deals with the etiology of disease and predicts the disease occurrence. It is also involved in evaluating the prevention and control of disease. Applied epidemiology deals with control of the disease and its distribution. So briefly, descriptive and analytic epidemiologies have two different aims. Two different types of studies done in epidemiology are given in Table 18.1.

Table 18.1: Differences between descriptive and analytic studies

Descriptive	Analytic
Describes nature and occurrence of disease	Deals with observational (cohort, case control, cross-sectional, ecologic study) or experimental (RCT, quasi experiment)– researcher assigns intervention (treatment), and estimates and tests its effect on health outcome

Measure of Disease Frequency

Cumulative Incidence

This is a measure of frequency, during a period of time.

Cumulative incidence = Number of new cases over a time/population at risk

This indicates the risk of the disease in a population at risk over a time. The values vary from 0 to 1.

Incidence Rate

Incidence rate is the number of new cases per population at risk in a given time.

Incidence rate = number of new cases of a time/person time at risk.

This indicates the speed of disease in the population over a time period and the values vary from zero to infinity.

Point Prevalence

This is the number of persons with disease at a given point interval divided by total number of persons in population.

Point prevalence = number of old and new vases at given point interval/total population

This indicates burden of disease and values vary from zero to one.

Evidence-Based Medicine (EBM)

EBM is an approach to practicing medicine in which the clinician is aware of the evidence in support of his/her clinical practice, and the strength of that evidence.

Evidence-based healthcare promotes the collection, interpretation, and integration of valid, important and applicable patient-reported, clinician-observed and research derived evidence. The best available evidence, moderated by patient circumstances and preferences, is applied to improve the quality of clinical judgements and facilitate effective healthcare.

A clinical experience is vital for treating patients but experience alone could be a problematic thing as today's experience could be tomorrow's mistake when the evidence changes. Rational treatment is going to stay. That is why understanding evidence-based medicine is important (Fig. 18.1). Table 18.2

Table 18.2: Levels of evidence

- **Level I:** Meta analysis of randomized control trials
- **Level II:** Large, well-designed randomized control trials
- **Level III:** Case control and cohort studies
- **Level IV:** Case reports and case series
- **Level V:** Expert opinion

gives different levels of medicine used in evidence-based medicine.

Medical Journals

Publication is the essence of science and doctors need to make the best possible decisions for patients. Medical journals are best tools to disseminate the knowledge among themselves and among peers. There are 20,000 print journals still EBM is not universally practiced and there is scope to do more.

Weakness of Published Literature

Many of the published studies may not be relevant. This is because they may not be upstream to clinical decisions being made, e.g. animal or *in vitro* studies. Also at times, the study populations/study settings do not reflect question type, practice population and settings. They may not be reliable as the study design may be poor, there may be bias and confounding, and there could be issues with validity and power of the study may not be sufficient.

Study Power

The ability of the study to detect an effect if in truth there is an effect.

A clinical trial may be underpowered if the duration is too short (too few events) or it includes too few people (too few events). So if the sample size is too small; power of the study to detect the wanted difference may be undermined. The study may also be undermined if the wrong outcome was used (too few events).

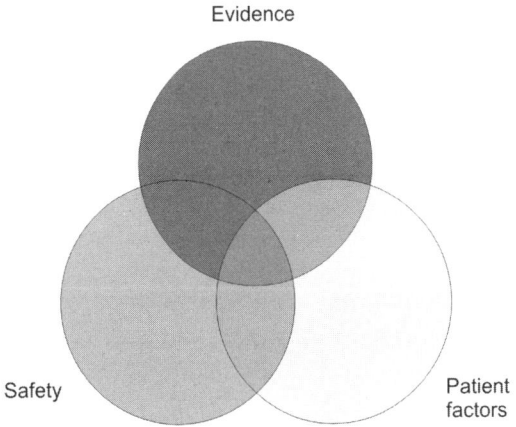

Fig. 18.1: Triad of evidence-based medicine

Expecting a higher level of statistical proof than is realistic for the condition and the intervention being tested could result in interpretation error. The chance of a natural error in research (called probability) is 1 in 20 (0.05). The chance of such an error (type I) = >1 in 20 (0.051) = not significant and the probability of making such an error to the tune of < 1 in 20 (0.049) = statistically significant.

Confidence Intervals

Confidence interval is an interval of values computed from the sample, that is almost sure to cover the true population value. It is important to know that we make confidence intervals using values computed from the sample, not the known values from the population. Confidence interval implies that in the 95% of the samples we take, the true population proportion (or mean) will be in the interval. This is also the same as saying we are 95% confident that the true population proportion (or mean) will be in the interval.

Bibliography

1. Clinical epidemiology and healthcare. http://ihpme.utoronto.ca/academics/rd/cehcr-mscphd/ (Downloaded online on February 8th 2017).

2. Clinical epidemiology and research methods. https://www.med.unc.edu/infdis/malawi/training/introduction-to-clinical-epidemiology-and-quantitative-research-methods (Downloaded online on February 8th 2017).

3. Introduction to epidemiology. https://onlinecourses.science.psu.edu/stat507/book/export/html/2 (Downloaded online on February 8th 2017).

Basic Statistical Tools in Medical Research

Learning objectives

Statistics is a *Latin* word, *status*, and it deals with collection, analysis and interpretation of data. Using *statistics* is alien to most of the doctors and is an ignored area. Present chapter deals with an overview of the same.

Statistics is the science of collecting, organizing, analyzing, and interpreting data in order to make decisions. The population is the collection of *all* outcomes, responses, measurement, or counts that are of interest.

A sample is the subset of a population. A parameter is a numerical description of a *population* characteristic.

Medical statistics deal with applications of statistics to medicine and the health sciences, including epidemiology, public health, forensic medicine, and clinical research. Medical statistics has been a recognized branch of statistics in the UK for more than 40 years but the term does not appear to have come into general use in North America, where the wider term 'biostatistics' is more commonly used.

There are several reasons, e.g. studying statistics is the basic requirement of medical research. Also one would have to update medical knowledge and this needs statistical information. For any kind of data management; good deal of information on medical statistics is needed.

History of Medical Statistics

In the year, 1929 a paper on application of statistics was published in physiology journal by Dunn. In later years, more than a dozen articles on statistical methods by Bradford Hill were published in the form of a book. In the middle of 20th century, a randomized trial of streptomycin for pulmonary tuberculosis was published. Since then the growth of statistics in medicine from has been tremendous. In India, the term "biostatistics" is used more often; however, with growth of medical research, the term "medical statistics" will find greater acceptance.

Understanding statistics is vital and without proper understanding and appreciation of medical statistics, the research may appear directionless, elusive and even misleading.

The data in medical statistics consists of information coming from observations, counts, measurements, or responses, etc. this information has to be analyzed to make proper sense. The data could be of two types (Table 19.1). Various types of data in statistics are given below.

a. *Nominal data*: Names are nominal data. Yes no responses could be another example.

b. *Ordinal*: They deal with order or severity like mild, moderate or severe.

c. *Interval data*: If the interval between values has an interpretation, this is an interval data, e.g. blood pressure: normal range is 120/80; the difference is meaningful.

d. *Ratio data*: This has absolute zero and the data can be multiplied or divided. Interval and ratio data are the highest form of data.

Table 19.1: Types of data

Qualitative data	Quantitative data
Non numerical entities, e.g. yes, no, names, etc.	Numerical measurements or counts
Usually descriptive in nature	Inferences can be drawn
Open-ended questionnaire, unstructured interviews or observations are tools used to collect data	Tests of significance are used
Analysis difficult	Analysis easy as several tests are employed

Variables

A variable is basically any character, number of quantity that can be measured or counted. Age, sex, weight, height are some of the examples of variables.

Variables can be classified as independent or dependent. An independent variable is the variable that is assumed to affect the influence outcome measure. A dependent variable is the variable that is dependent on or influenced by the independent variable(s). A dependent variable is the variable under measurement. On the other hand an independent variable is the variable that can predict. For example, if we are trying to measure heart rate variability among medical students during examination time; and trying to predict the effect of examination stress on the same, then heart rate is our dependent variable and stress is independent.

Intervening Variable

In simple words, an intervening variable is the variable that links the independent and dependent variable. For example, in a study of occupation and education; the income level can work as an intervening variable. This is also called a mediating variable that may be used to explain causal link between other variables.

Parameter is usually presented by Greek letters such as μ, π, σ, etc. The parameters in research are unknown and to know the parameter of a population. We need a sample to be able to do so (*see* below).

Research Designs

Selecting the appropriate statistical test requires several steps. Test selection should be based on what is the goal of doing the analysis, like is it description of the data or comparison of values or prediction about an association, etc. Alternatively, the goal can be to quantify or prove the effectiveness of the drug. Proving causality could be another aim.

One has to look as to what kind of data has been collected. Also, one should determine if the data is normally distributed or not. One can use parametric or non-parametric test. Q–q plots, histogram, stem and leaf plots are some of the common methods of knowing about the normality of data. Kolmogorov-Smirnov test is a popular statistical test for the same.

Before choosing the test, one has to know as to what are the assumptions of the statistical test one would like to use. If those have been sorted then one should determine if the collected data meets these assumptions.

Obviously, there are various assumptions for each test. Before one selects a test, one should be sure to check the assumptions of each test. Before starting up the project, it is needed that one consults a statistician or review statistical/research methods with some consultant.

Some examples of common assumptions of the statistical tests are:

a. The dependent variable will need to be measured on a certain level, e.g. interval level.

b. The independent variable(s) will need to be measured on a certain level, e.g. ordinal level.

c. The population is normally distributed (not skewed).

If the data does not meet the assumptions for a specific test, you may be able to use a non-parametric test instead.

Epidemiology Aims

Epidemiology aims to measure disease frequency, and quantify disease. It is also aimed at assessing the distribution of disease. It eventually aims to answer further questions like who is getting disease, where is the disease occurring, when is the disease occurring, formulation of hypotheses concerning causal and preventive factors, etc. It should also identify determinants of disease. Note that hypotheses are tested using epidemiologic studies.

Study types

a. *Descriptive studies*: These are aimed to describe occurrence of outcome.
b. *Analytic studies*: Analytic studies describe association between exposure and outcome.

The details of other study types are given along with the respective chapters.

Dealing with Statistician

This is a very important question for students in biomedical sciences. To guide the design of an experiment or survey prior to data collection; it is important that we consult the statistician before starting the treatment. The statistician can help analyze the data using proper statistical procedures and techniques. This can help to present and interpret the results to researchers and other decision makers in a form that is easily understood.

This is one of the most common questions that confront medical students. This is a perplexing situation when guide tells, "Go and talk to statistician" and student feels, "What do I need to ask him or her apart from the fact that I have to get sample size calculated for thesis?"

Now, in a statistician's chamber a student is asked the following:

a. What is the research question?
b. What is the hypothesis?
c. What amount of alpha error is acceptable?
d. How much beta error one wants?
e. What is sampling method?
f. What precision is acceptable?

These are some of the difficult questions that a student has to answer. Some of them can be helped by statistician but he/she cannot provide answer to all of them. So one would have to be prepared to answer them clearly and coherently; if one were to get best out of statistician. The text given below is expected to provide answer to these questions. This can be approached via alpha-beta A, B, C, D, E, F.

A: This is called **alpha error** (type 1 error). This is the chance that a mistake that we shall make once we start our study. This is when we draw "wrong conclusions" about the significance be it clinical or statistically. That means, we may have incorrect rejection of null hypothesis (false positive).

B: This is **beta error** or the ability to pick up the difference when it was there but we could not spot it. This is when we miss out on things. It could be serious, as you know, something that was there but we could not pick it up. This means, we may incorrectly retain a null hypothesis (false negative).

C: Confidence level is the confidence that a researcher will have in the finding or the variable of interest in the given confidence interval. It is expressed as a percentage and shows how often true result of the population who would pick and answer lies with the confidence interval. For example, if the confidence level if 95%, which most researchers are; then it means one is 95% certain of finding the truth within confidence interval.

This should be differentiated from confidence interval is the range in which the variable of interest is likely to lie. This is a given range in which the population parameter has to lie. Generally, it is set at 5%. It is also called precision. That means, one would want to be as precise as possible. If more precision is needed then one could set it at 1% level. This should be differentiated from *p-value* or level of significance. We set this level before the study begins and state, "The probability that we may go wrong is 1:20, i.e. there is a 5% chance that we may accept results as significant even when they are not!" Similarly, another kind of error can error can also creep in! To be able to detect this difference when it actually exists is called "power of study".

D: Deviation (standard deviation): One should have some idea of the standard deviation that is present in the variable of interest. If no such data exists, one can calculate the same using a pilot study. Standard deviation is represented by the Greek letter sigma ó or the Latin letter s. It is a measure that can be used to quantify amount of variation or dispersion in a set of data.

E: Effect size is the medically or clinically relevant difference that one would consider as significant. In many of the statistical parameters described above, if not most of these, statisticians will offer limited help. This is because; these variables are determined by researcher.

How big is the sample size one would need in the research is a common question. An adequate sample size with good power is the key to successful outcome of study.

Variables

There are two kinds of variables that we deal within statistics: *dependent* and *independent*. *Dependent variable* is also called *outcome variable* and is the variable under measurement. *Independent variable* is the one that cannot be manipulated.

Data

Data is made-up of *Latin* word, *datum*, which means a variable under study. For example, height, weight, blood pressure is various types of data. This is also called variables, characters or attributes. These can be discrete if they take-up one value or continuous if they could take any value. For example, number of students in a class is a discrete value. On the other hand, if we take height of doctors working in cardiology unit; this is a continuous variable. That means, if we take height in meters, inches, centimeters, or millimeters; some change may be seen.

So far we have spoken about the types of data. But what is data? Webster's International

Dictionary defines *data* as a numerical value. So, this is basically statistics is a science dealing with the collection, analysis, interpretation, and presentation of data.

Statistics as a science and art aims at dealing with variation in data through collection, classification, and analysis in such a way as to obtain reliable results that could be extrapolated. The statistics could be descriptive or inferential (Table 19.2).

Table 19.2: Features of two major types of statistics

Descriptive	Inferential
Organization, summation and data display using graphs and charts	Statistical data analysis to estimate the value of a population parameter from the characteristics of a sample
Aim is to explore the data and to describe a phenomena/character	Aim is to draw valid conclusions

Types of Statistics

Broadly, there are two types of statistics: *Observational* and *experimental*. Observational is could be descriptive or analytical. Descriptive is also called qualitative and quantitative.

Descriptive statistics deals with qualitative data like male and female, tall and short, thin and fat, etc. and the experimental deals with something that is measured with accuracy.

Qualitative data is used to describe a phenomenon in clinical studies while quantitative data is of higher order and is used make inferences regarding interventions using statistical analysis. Studies types are given in Table 19.3.

Table 19.3: Studies type
- Qualitative
  - Describe → form categories (categorical)
- Quantitative → continuous
  - Measure → infer
    - So descriptive and inferential

Population and Sample

Population is the universe that could be studied while sample is a small part of the same. Study population is the part of whole population: The whole collection of individuals that one intends to study is called study universe. A sample is a representative part of the population. It is important to know that the randomization is an indispensible way to make the sample representative (Fig. 19.1).

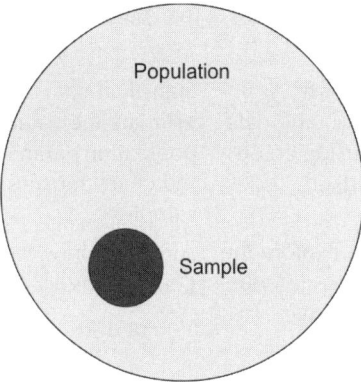

Fig. 19.1: Analogy to explain relationship between population and sample. Sample is a small part of the population. Our aim is to draw valid conclusions from this sample that could be extrapolated to entire population

Alpha Level

Alpha level, or significance level, is the value that is determined by the researcher in order to accept or reject the null hypothesis. It is a pre-determined value before the study begins and is not a calculated one. In other words, if we select a value of 0.05, findings would be deemed statistically significant if they were found to be 0.05 or less.

Alpha levels indicates the probability that the null hypothesis will be rejected when it is true. In other words, if the null hypothesis is wrongly rejected, this is called type 1 error or alpha error.

For example, in a trial of new drug X, the null hypothesis might be that the new drug A is no better than the current drug B.

H_0: There is no difference between drug A and B.

Type 1 Error

A type 1 error would occur if we concluded that the two drugs produced different effects when there was no difference between them. This can produce a gross error as the drug without efficacy could be introduced clinically.

Type 2 Error

Beta is the probability of making a type 2 error when testing a hypothesis. Type 2 error is failing to detect an association when one exists, or failing to reject the null hypothesis when it is actually false. Errors in hypothesis testing are given in Table 19.4.

You kept the null hypothesis when you should not have. If drug A and drug B produced different efficacy, it could be concluded that they produce the same effects. Some errors of hypothesis testing are given in Table 19.4.

Table 19.4: Errors in hypothesis testing		
Reject null	*Do not reject*	
Null hypothesis	Type 1 error	Correct decision
Alternative hypothesis	Correct decision	Type 2 error

Sampling

Sampling is among the trickiest part of medical research. A correctly collected sample is the key to hypothesis testing or describing a phenomena. The preferred type of sampling is random: Random is by chance! The random event is the event may occur or may not occur in one experiment. Before the experiment, nobody is sure whether the event will occur or not. Examples of random events include weather, traffic accidents, etc.

a. *Systematic random sampling*: This is a common way of selecting sample. The subjects are sampled at regular interval starting from a random number. For example, every 3rd or 4th person could be chosen.

b. *Stratified sampling*: This kind of sampling has members from each segment of the population. This ensures that each segment has been represented.

c. *Cluster sample*: This has all the members from randomly selected segment of population. Members are selected from different geographical areas "clusters". All members in each selected groups could be used.

d. *Convenience sampling*: This involves only of available members of the population.

Sampling Error

Sampling error is the error arising due to the difference between observed value and true value.

Several types of error can error in sampling. The statistics of different samples from same population could be different from each other! That means sampling has not been done properly. The statistics could be different from the parameter! The sampling error exists in any research. Sampling error may not be avoidable but may be estimated.

Methods of Presenting Data

There are various methods of presenting data in clinical trials/medical research (Table 19.5, Figs 19.2, 19.3 and 19.4). Most of them are done before analysis.

Table 19.5: Common methods of data presentations

- Stem and leaf plot
- Histogram
- Bar chart
- Dot plot
- Scatter plot

Stem and leaf plot (Table 19.6)

Stem and leaf plots are a method of showing frequency with which certain classes of value occur. Make a frequency distribution or histogram of values and then one can use the stem-and-leaf plot.

For example, given is the number of marks that students scored in their mid-term MD examination in Radiology out of 50. Values are: 12, 13, 21, 27, 33, 34, 35, 37, 40, 40, 41.

We could make a frequency distribution table showing how many tens, twenties, thirties, and forties we have.

Frequency class	Frequency
10–19	2
20–29	2
30–39	4
40–49	3

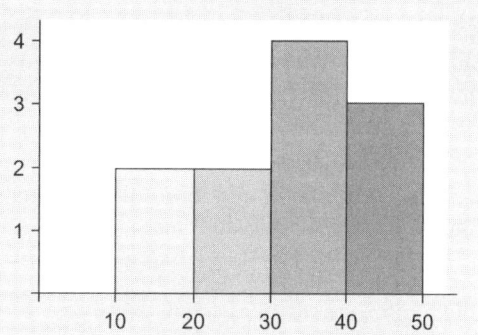

Fig. 19.2: Histogram of the data values

Table 19.6: Features of stem and leaf plot

- Useful in knowing shape of distribution
- Retains original data
- Also describes outliers
- Tells about mode
- Largest digits → stem, smallest → leaf

Stem	Leaf
1	2 3
2	1 7
3	3 4 5 7
4	0 0 1

The "stem" of the values is the left handed column containing 1 to 10 digits and "leaves" on the right hand side show all ones digits for tens, twenties, thirties, and forties. Horizontal leaves correspond to vertical bars in histogram and leaves have lengths that equal the number of frequency Table 19.7.

Table 19.7: Features of histogram

- Graphical distribution of tabulated frequencies
- Continuous data
- Numerical intervals of equal size
- Independent variable plotted along the horizontal axis and the dependent variable along the vertical axis

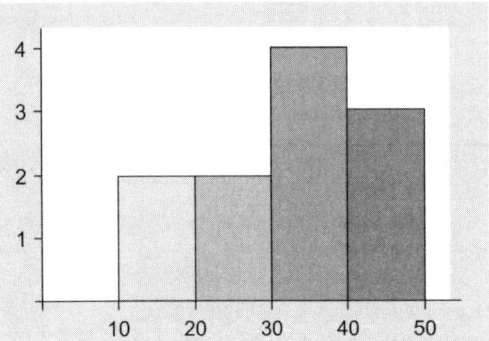

Fig. 19.3: Histogram of the number of marks that students scored in their mid-term MD examination in Radiology out of 50. Values are: 12, 13, 21, 27, 33, 34, 35, 37, 40, 40, 41

Table 19.8: Features of bar chat

- >200 years old
- Used for categorical data
- One axis shows categories, another shows values
- Could be horizontal or vertical
- Spaces between values → bar, no space → histogram

Dot Plots

This is a graphical depiction of data using dots. This is a very simple representation (Table 19.9).

Table 19.9: Features of dot plot

- Dots plotted on a simple scale
  - Described 100 years back as a hand drawn graph
- Used for moderate size data
- Mostly for continuous data
- Clusters, gaps and outliers can be highlighted

Box and whisker plot and inter-quartile range:
On a scale, one has to take lowest and highest value (Fig. 19.5). Then divide it into quarters of equal size say Q1, Q2, Q3, Q4 as shown below.

Following is the number of marks of MBBS students in pharmacology practical exercises:

4, 17, 7, 14, 18, 12, 3, 16, 10, 4, 4, 11

Arrange them in ascending order:

3, 4, 4, 4, 7, 10, 11, 12, 14, 16, 17, 18

Divide them into 4 quartiles:

3, 4, 4, 4, 7, 1011, 12, 14, 16, 17, 18

Calculate: Q1, Q2, and Q3:

Q1 = 4 + 4/2 = 4
Q2 = 10 + 11 = 21/2 = 11.5
Q3 = 14 + 16 = 30/2 = 15

Inter-quartile range: Q3 − Q1 = 15 − 4 = 11

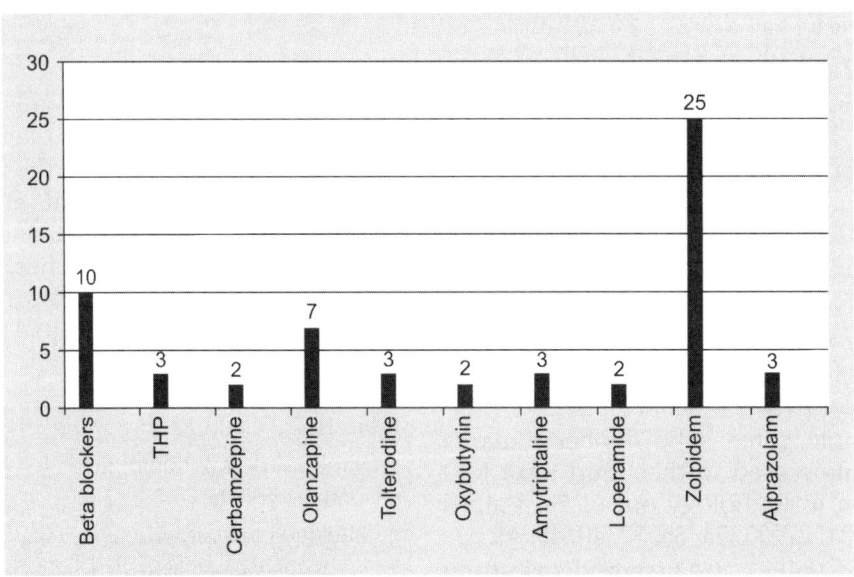

Fig. 19.4: Bar chart showing the use of drugs distribution of drugs having the potential to cause cognitive impairment and the number of patients taking them (Dhikav, et al, 2014)

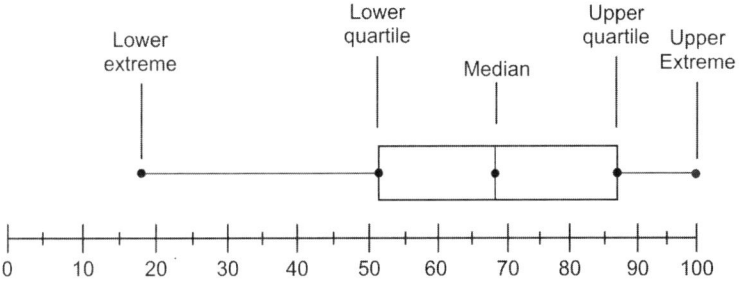

Fig. 19.5: Box and whisker plot. This depicts data via quartiles. Plot tells us about spread, skewness and outliers. May look primitive compared to histogram but has advantage of knowing about data distribution

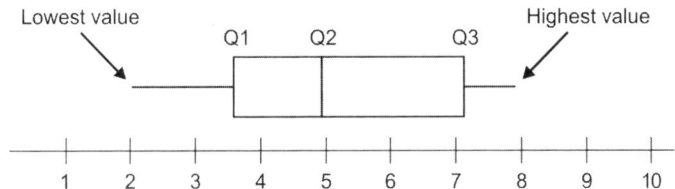

Fig. 19.6: Box and whisker plot and inter-quartile range

Data Distribution and Tests of Normality

How do we know that our data is normally distributed?

Normal Distribution

Normal distribution (Fig. 19.7) in probability theory is the most commonly occurring continuous probability distribution. This will tell that most value will fall between 3 standard deviations around mean. Data can get distributed towards left or right but in most cases; it tends to have a bell shaped curve (normal distribution).

If the data is normally distributed; approximately 2/3 (68%) of values are within

1 standard deviation of the mean, 95% of values are within 2 standard deviations of the mean and 99% of values are within 3 standard deviations of the mean.

It is important to know data distribution right from beginning so that we proceed with statistical tests in an appropriate way. There are different tests for different types of data (Table 19.10).

- In descriptive data
  - Goodness of fit
- Inferential statistics
  - Null hypothesis

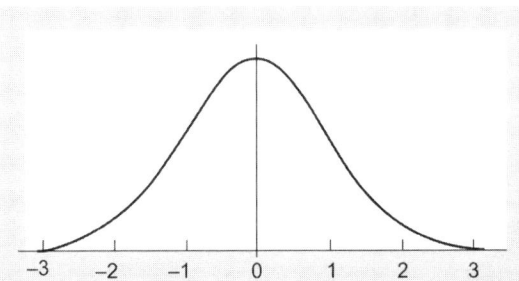

Fig. 19.7: Normal distribution. Most values are concentrated around the mean

Table 19.10: Type of data and test we use for knowing type of distribution

- Descriptive statistics
  - Histogram
  - Q–Q plot
  - Box and whisker plot
  - Kurtosis
- Inferential
  - Kolmogrov-smnirov test

Gross rules of thumb for normality of data
- When n is greater than 30, this is a good approximation to results from more sensitive tests.
- If the standard deviation is more than 3 points from mean, question normality of data.

Methods of Dispersion

Most of the summary measures deal with mean, median and mode and provide a measure of central tendency. However, they fail to tell anything about the data spread. So therefore, more measures are needed to know what is the extent of data spread (Table 19.11).

Table 19.11: Data dispersion indicators
- Range
- Standard deviation
- Absolute mean deviation
- Coefficient of variation

Variance

Average squared deviation from mean is called variance (S^2). It has limited value nowadays and used more commonly. It tells about spread out of data from their means.

It is calculated by:

$$S^2 = \frac{\Sigma(X - \bar{X})^2}{n-1}$$

S^2 = Variance

One has to square the differences of the individual values from the mean to get rid of negative sign. Then sum them up and divide them by $n-1$. Why $n-1$? This is because; we are taking one sample from the population.

A simple formula for variance can be given as:

$$\text{Variance} = \frac{\Sigma x^2}{N}$$

Where,
x is the deviation of the value from the mean, i.e. $X - \bar{X}$
N is the total number of values.

Standard Error (SE)

This is often called standard deviation of the sampling distribution. It can be used, both for means and medians. Both standard deviation and standard error may get used interchangeably. However, they are different. Standard deviation tells about variability of data and hence spread. It can be shown that 95% of observations lie within 2 standard deviations. Standard error is the accuracy with which data represents population measures the accuracy with which sample mean deviates from actual mean.

Smaller the standard error; more representative the sample will be of the overall population. That means, standard error is inversely proportional to the sample size. In gross terms, it means how far is the sample mean from the population means.

$$SE = \frac{SD}{\sqrt{(n)}}$$

Skewed Data

Skewed data means, it tends to have a longish tail on one side or the other. It can be positive, or negative. Figure 19.8 details various types of skewed distributions.

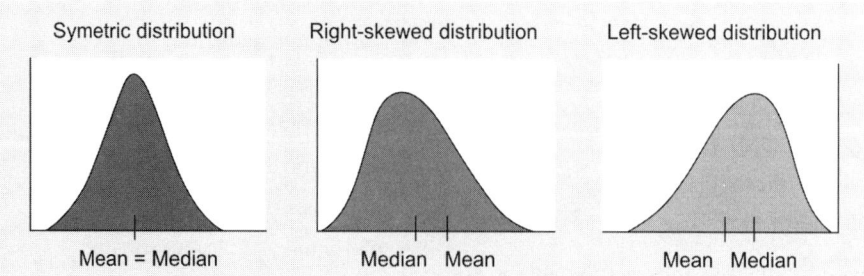

Fig. 19.8: Various types of skewed distributions

How to calculate Pearson's coefficient of skewness:
- Subtract mean from median
- Multiply by 3
- And divide by standard deviation
- Value ranges from −1 to +1
- < − 1 means left skewness
- > + 1 means right skewness.

Coefficient of Variation
- CV = SD/mean × 100
- Tells about percentage of deviation from mean.

Standard Deviation (SD)

Average distance of scores from the mean can be calculated from standard deviation. This is most often done using standard deviation. It is the most common measure of dispersion or variability of data set.

It is calculated as square root of the mean. It depicts average deviation from mean and is expressed in same units as data. This is unlike variance that is expressed as square root. This may artificially inflate dispersion.

Standard deviation helps in calculating confidence interval. A low SD indicates data is close to its mean, while high SD indicates data is far from mean. *Chebyshev rule* says that 3/4 of data within 2 standard deviations.

Importance of Standard Deviation

Distribution along the normal curve can be known if we know about the standard deviation. A small standard deviation (Fig. 19.9) will mean that the distance from the mean of the dataset is small and is very close to the mean. A large dataset however may mean there may be an outlier or the data is skewed. That means, variance of this data is more.

For example, in a routine assessment of students in a class, if the average score on a test was 80 and the standard deviation was just 2, the scores would be more clustered around the mean than if the standard deviation was 10.

How to Calculate Standard Deviation?

Formula for calculation of standard deviation is given below:

$$S = \sqrt{\frac{\Sigma(X - M)^2}{n-1}}$$

S = Standard deviation
Σ = Sum of
X = Individual scores
M = Mean of all scores
n = Sample size (number of scores)

An organized chart will help us calculate the standard deviation easily.

One should first take all the values, and then take the arithmetic mean; then keep subtracting the individual values from the mean. Ignore the negative sign. A simple example has been given below.

Dataset: 1, 2, 3, 4, 5, 6, 7, 8, 9, 10

Arithmetic mean = 1 + 2 + 3 + 4 + 5 + 6 + 7 + 8 + 9 +10 = 55/10 = 5.5

Standard deviation =
1–5.5 = −4.5
2–5.5 = −3.5
3–5.5 = −2.5
4–5.5 = −1.5
5–5.5 = −0.5
6–5.5 = 0.5
7–5.5 = 2.5
8–5.5 = 3.5
9–5.5 = 4.5
10–5.5 = 4.5

- **SD = 2.8 ± 1.49**

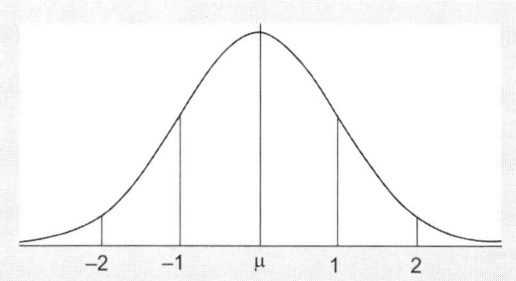

Fig. 19.9. The normal curve. Standard deviation is a constant interval from the mean

Keep few points in mind while calculating standard deviation:

a. Purpose of squaring the differences is to rule out the negative sign so that the differences do not become neutralized.

b. n–1 is used because we are calculating the standard deviation for a sample and not for the entire population. Had it been for entire population, then we can calculate it using N and not n–1.

c. Completing the calculation:

$$S = \sqrt{\frac{\Sigma(X - M)^2}{n - 1}}$$

Divide total squared deviations by n–1. That leaves 10/4. Take the square root of 2.5. The standard deviation equals 1.58.

Mean

Mean is the most common measure of variability among the dataset if it is reported with standard deviation and the confidence interval, another measure of variability in dataset.

Median

In statistics and probability theory, the median is a measure of central tendency that separates one half of the data from the other, i.e. middle value.

If observations of a variable are arranged in ascending and descending ordered, then the median corresponds to the middle observation. The median value corresponds to a cumulative percentage of 50% (i.e. 50% of the values are below the median and 50% of the values are above the median). The position of the median is $\{(n + 1) \div 2\}^{th}$ **value**, where n is the number of values in a set of data.

In order to calculate the median, the data must first be ranked sorted in ascending order or descending order. The median is the number in the middle. If there are two middle values; then both are added and divided by 2.

Mode

This is most frequently occurring value.

Calculate mode of the following from the mini mental state score of dementia patients: 22, 21, 22, 20, 23, 23, 22, 22, 22, 24, 27, 27, 29, 30, 22

Mode is most frequently occurring value: 22.

Confidence Interval

Nowadays it is becoming almost customary to report the values of confidence interval along with mean and standard deviation.

Put simply, if someone says that on a cloudy day; what is the possibility of rains in Delhi? The possibility naturally will be predictably high. But how sure are you about this probability? One has to give a range, i.e. 60–80%. Real value will lie between this.

So confidence interval is a very important measure of variability and can help us in knowing what is the likelihood of the value of the data being same if the study were to be repeated by someone else somewhere. Two or more means can also be compared using confidence intervals.

What is Sample Size?

Sample size is the requirement of the number of subjects to assure a given probability of detecting a statistically significant effect of a given magnitude if one truly exists? Naturally, to be able to draw valid conclusions, adequate sample size is a must. Details of sample size calculations are described elsewhere.

Why do Sample Size Calculation?

Sample size calculation is crucial for medical research. One cannot be sure if one has made the right decision regarding the effect of the intervention until and unless the right sample size has been included. However, we want *enough* subjects enrolled to adequately address study question to feel comfortable that we have reached correct conclusion. Naturally, if cannot adequately address study question. The time, discomfort and risk to subjects have served no purpose.

The study may conclude no effect of an intervention that is beneficial. If that happens, naturally the current and future subjects may not benefit from new intervention based on current (inconclusive) study.

Now, if one has too many subjects in the study, then unnecessarily they would be exposed to the risk. Naturally, one should enroll only enough patients to answer study question, to minimize the discomfort and risk subjects may be exposed to.

Study Hypothesis

There are two kinds of hypothesis:

a. **Null hypothesis (H_0):** Means, no difference between groups; mathematically:

$H_0: p_1 = p_2$ $\qquad$ $H_0: m_1 = m_2$

b. **Alternative hypothesis (H_A):** There is a difference between groups; mathematically:

$H_A: p_1 {}^1 p_2$ $\qquad$ $H_A: m_1 {}^1 m_2$

Probability Value

Probability value is the chance of obtaining observed result or one more extreme value when groups are equal (under null hypothesis or H_0).

Test of significance for the null hypothesis (H_0)

Based on distribution of a test statistic assuming H_0 is true; the probability value below 0.05 in medical research means, alternative hypothesis can be accepted. It should be noted that it is not the probability that H_0 is true.

Delta (Δ) is the measure of true population difference that must be estimated. Or in other words, it is the difference of medical importance; mathematically:

$$\Delta = |p_1 - p_2| \quad \Delta = |m_1 - m_2|$$

Errors in Hypothesis Testing

Type 1 error occurs when rejecting H_0 when H_0 is true; it is denoted by alpha (α) or the type 1 error rate. It also indicates the maximum *p-value* that is considered statistically significant.

Type 2 error occurs when one fails to reject H_0 when H_0 is false and is detonated by β or the type 2 error rate. The quantities such as α, β, Δ and N are all interrelated. Holding all other values constant, what happens to the power of the study if:

- Effect size (Δ) increases? $\qquad$ Power ↑
- Alpha α decreases? $\qquad$ Power ↑
- Sample size (N) increases? $\quad$ Power ↑
- Variability increases? $\qquad$ Power ↑

Typical error rates are kept as $\alpha = .05$ and $\beta = 0.1$ or 0.2 (80 or 90% power).

Study Power

Power $(1 - \beta)$ is the probability of detecting group effect given the size of the effect size of medically relevant difference (Δ) and the sample size of the trial (N).

So in other words, the power of a study deals with the fact that if a limited number of subjects are available; what is the likelihood of finding a statistically significant effect of a given magnitude if one truly exists?

Sample Size Calculation

Note that the sample size very sensitive to values of effect size (Δ). Large N required for high power to detect small differences and *vice versa*. Therefore, while planning a study one should consider the current knowledge and feasibility.

To compare two means from two different independent samples, i.e.

$H_0: \mu_1 = \mu_2$ we would need the following:

α level

β level $(1 - \text{power})$

Expected population difference ($\Delta = |\mu_1 - \mu_2|$)

Expected population standard deviation (σ_1, σ_2)

There are two approaches to sample size calculations:

a. **Precision-based:** One would have to decide as to with what precision does one want to estimate the proportion, mean difference, etc. Suppose if one want to estimate unknown parameter with a certain degree of precision. What you are essentially saying is that you want your confidence interval to be a certain width.

In general a 95% confidence interval is given by the formula:

Estimate ± 2(approx)1 × standard error (SE), where SE is the standard error of whatever one is estimating. This is because 95% confidence intervals are usually based on the normal distribution or a t-distribution—for a normal distribution the value is 1.96; for t-distributions the value is generally just over 2.

$$P = \pm Z_{CI}\sigma_{\bar{X}}$$

$$\Rightarrow P = \pm Z_{CI}\frac{\sigma_{\bar{X}}}{\sqrt{n}}$$

Therefore, sample size will be:

$$\Rightarrow n = \frac{Z_{CI}^2 \ \sigma^2}{P^2}$$

Where, P is precision, Z = standard normal deviate, sigma = standard deviation, CI = confidence internal, n = sample size.

b. **Power-based:** This is another way in which the sample size gets calculated. One would have to decide as to how small a difference is it important to be detected and with what degree of certainty?

The formula for any standard error always contains n, the sample size. Therefore, if you specify the width of the 95% confidence interval, you have a formula that you can solve to find n. Suppose one wishes to carry out a trial of a new antihypertensives among the aged between 50 and 60.

One randomly selected some subjects for this purpose. Some (n) of these receive the new treatment and others (n) receive the standard treatment, then one would measure each subject's systolic blood pressure as a dependent variable.

Comparing the mean blood pressure in the two groups is done using unpaired t-test and calculating a 95% confidence interval for the true difference in means.

One would like 95% confidence interval to have width of 10 mm Hg (i.e. one wants to be 95% sure that the true difference in means is within ± 5 mm Hg of your estimated difference

in means). Now, the question is how many subjects will you need to include in your study? The sample size formula is given below:

Sample size formula for percentages (nominal or ordinal)

$$n = \frac{Z^2 \times ([P \times Q])}{e^2}$$

Where,

n = Required sample size

Z = The Z value for your desired confidence level

P = Estimation of the population %

Q = (100 − P)

e = Desired accuracy range

Degrees of Freedom

This represents the number of independent observations in a sample. Degrees of freedom is a measure that states the number of variables that can change within a statistical test. This is calculated by $n-1$ (sample size − 1). Degrees of freedom is determined by the researcher and is denoted by α. Importantly, this is affected by the sample size and the nature of the experiment.

Critical Value

Critical value is a probability table value and is used to know the level of significance. One has to first determine degrees of freedom. Before finding the critical value; one has to decide the level of significance for which the critical value needs to be found. If the calculated value of t is less than the critical value of t obtained from the table, the null hypothesis is not rejected. If the calculated value of t is greater than the critical value of t from the table, the null hypothesis is rejected.

Common levels of significance at which the critical values are checked are: 0.05, 0.01, 0.001. Critical values indicate the probability that the researcher made an error in rejecting the null hypothesis. Common tests used in hypothesis testing are given in Table 19.12.

Table 19.12: Parameteric vs nonparametric tests

Parametric	Non parametric
t-test	Mann-whitney test
ANOVA	Kruskal-wallis test
Pearson's correlation coefficient	Chi-square test
Regression analysis	Wilcoxon test

Parametric Tests

Parametric tests assume that the variable in question is from a normal distribution. Non-parametric tests do not require the assumption of normality. Most non-parametric tests do not require an interval or ratio level of measurement; can be used with nominal/ordinal level data.

Nonparametric Tests

Use when all assumptions of parametric statistics cannot be met. Nonparameteric tests can be used with data that are not normally distributed.

Univariate Analysis

Univariate analysis is the analysis of one variable.

Bivariate Analysis

Bivariate analysis is a kind of data analysis that explores the association between two variables. Some examples of bivariate analysis include: Pearson's correlation, Spearman's Rho, etc.

Multivariate Analysis

Multivariate analysis is the analysis of more than two variables. Some examples of multivariate analysis include multiple regression analysis, multiple logistic regressions.

Chi-Squared Test

Chi-square test is often used for testing significance of patterns in qualitative data. The test statistic is based on counts that represent the number of items that fall in each category. Test statistics measures the agreement between actual counts and expected counts assuming the null hypothesis.

The *chi-square* distribution can be used to see whether or not an observed counts agree with an expected counts.

O = Observed count and

E = Expected count

$$x^2 = \Sigma \frac{(O - E)^2}{E}$$

The most obvious difference between the *chi-square* tests and the other hypothesis tests, e.g. *t* and ANOVA, etc. is the nature of the data. For *chi-square*, the data are frequencies rather than numerical scores.

The *chi-square* test for goodness-of-fit uses frequency data from a sample to test hypotheses about the shape or proportions of a population. Each individual in the sample is classified into one category on the scale of measurement. The data, called observed frequencies, simply count how many individuals from the sample are in each category.

The second *chi-square* test, the *chi-square* test for independence, can be used and interpreted in two different ways:

a. Testing hypotheses about the relationship between two variables in a population.
b. Testing hypotheses about differences between proportions for two or more populations.

Although the two versions of the test for independence appear to be different, they are equivalent and they are interchangeable.

Mann Whitney *U* Test

Mann Whitney *U* Test is the nonparametric equivalent of the independent *t* test. It needs two independent groups. Ordinal measurement of the dependent variables are taken and the sampling distribution of *U* is known and is used to test hypotheses in the same way as the *t* distribution.

The Kruskal-Wallis Test

The Kruskal-Wallis test is a nonparametric procedure that can be used to compare more than two populations in a completely randomized design. All $n = n_1 + n_2 + \ldots + n_k$ measurements are jointly ranked (i.e. treat as one large sample). We use the sums of the ranks of the k samples to compare the distributions.

In this test, one would rank the total measurements in all k samples from 1 to n. Tied observations are assigned average of the ranks they would have gotten if not tied.

One would calculate T_i = rank sum for the ith sample i = 1, 2,..., k and then calculate the test statistic (Kruskal-Wallis H):

$$H = \frac{12}{n(n+1)} \Sigma \frac{T_i^2}{n_i} - 3(n+1)$$

H_0: The k distributions are identical versus
H_a: At least one distribution is different

When H_0 is true, the test statistic H has an approximate chi-square distribution with $df = k-1$. One would use a right-tailed rejection region or *p-value* based on the chi-square distribution.

PARAMETRIC TESTS

Student t-test

Student's t-test allows the comparison of the mean of 2 groups. This test compares actual difference between two means in relation to the variation in the data. This is expressed as the standard deviation of the difference between the means.

For example, if doctor X gives two different drugs to a group of diabetics to see if blood sugar lowering times differ, and if the difference between times are in fact significant.

The null hypothesis: Drug A and B will have equal blood sugar lowering times (no difference). The alternative hypothesis says the drug A and B will have different blood sugar lowering times.

Analysis of Variance (ANOVA)

Analysis of Variance (ANOVA) is a common test that allows the comparison of 3 or more groups. ANOVA looks at the variation within groups, then determines how that variation would translate into variation between groups (considering number of participants).

If observed differences are larger than what would be expected by chance, the findings are statistically significant.

Analysis of Covariance (ANCOVA)

This is a combination of ANOVA and regression together. ANCOVA can be used to compare treatments, after controlling for quantitative factor believed to be related to response unlike ANOVA where such a controlling cannot be done. This can also be used to compare regression equations among groups (e.g. common slopes and/or intercepts).

Correlation

This is a measure of relationship between two or more variables. This is mathematically expressed as *correlation coefficient* (Table 19.13). It can range between –1.00 to +1.00. The value of –1.00 represents a perfect negative correlation while a value of +1.00 represents a perfect positive correlation. A value of zero represents a lack of correlation (Fig. 19.10).

Table 19.13: How to interpret correlation coefficient (r)?

r = +1: Very strong, positive relationship

r = 0: No linear relationship between two variables (x) and (y)

r = –1: Very strong, but negative relationship, i.e. if (x) increases then (y) decreases

The most widely-used type of correlation coefficient is Pearson (r), also called linear or product-moment correlation.

Properties of correlation coefficient (r):
a. Pearson correlation (r) determines the extent to which values of the two variables are "proportional" to each other.

b. The value of correlation (i.e. correlation coefficient) does not depend on the specific measurement units used, e.g. the correlation between height and weight will be identical regardless of whether inches and pounds, or centimeters and kilograms are used as measurement units.

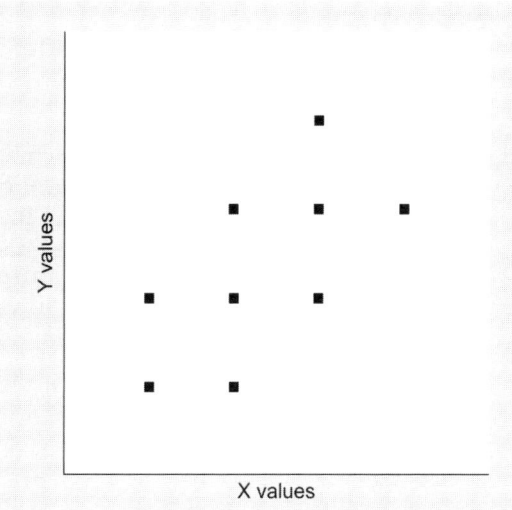

Fig. 19.10: Scatter-plot for correlation between left and right medial temporal lobe (Dhikav, et al, 2014). Pearson's correlation coefficient (r) between left and right medial lobe atrophy was calculated to be 0.45 and correlation coefficient (R^2) was 0.2. This suggests weak relationship between left and right. This was consistent with insignificant difference between left and right medial temporal lobe atrophy scores

c. Proportional means linearly related, i.e. correlation (r) is high if the dotes are mostly around the middle line and it can be shown by a straight line.

d. Even if the "strength or magnitude" of a correlation (r) is high; it is risky and inappropriate to assume that there is a causal or "cause-effect relationship" between the two variables. It just depicts a *strong* association.

e. Be aware of confounding variables as spurious associations may emerge. For example, if we do a study of vitamin D levels of the corporate employees in a big city as Delhi or Mumbai, then it might come out to be low. And if you ignore the influence of sunlight (a confounder) it with sunlight exposure there may not be a good correlation as employees spend lot of time inside the air-conditioned offices. That means, to get a good correlation, it is important to "control" extraneous influences.

f. At times, it may not be clearly known what the confounding variable is. In that case, results should be interpreted with caution. In such situations, we can do "partial correlation" when the confounder is hidden and is exhibiting a potential influence.

The middle line around which there could be many dotes is called the *regression line* or *least squares line* (related to regression analysis).

As mentioned above, the Pearson correlation coefficient (r) represents the linear relationship between two variables. If the correlation coefficient is squared, then the resulting r^2 value is R^2 (called the coefficient of determination).

R^2 and represents the proportion of common variation in the two variables (i.e. the "strength" or "magnitude" of the relationship between two variables).

Correlation allows an examination of the relationship between variables. Correlation asks if there is a relationship between these variables or not. If there is correlation then is it positive or negatively related.

Correlation coefficient value of 0 means that there is no relationship between the variables, a negative value (e.g. –1) means negative relationship, positive value (1.g. 1) means a positive relationship. It is important to know that presence of correlation is not a proof of causation. For example, if we want to know about the relationship between exercise and depression; then one can use correlation.

The question is: Does depression increase when the intensity of exercise increases? Or does depression decrease when the intensity of exercise increases?

Alternatively, is there no significant correlation between exercise and depression?

All such hypothesis can be tested using correlation analysis.

Regression

Linear regression focuses on prediction of the effect of one or more independent variables on the dependent variable. Regression involves the discovering of equation for a line that is the best fit for the given data. That linear equation is then used to predict values for the data. For example, if we want to know if A and B variables predict event C; then one can use regression.

This is also the analysis of relationship between two variables and the most common type is called as *regression analysis*. It could be of many types (Fig. 19.11):

    a. Linear regression
    b. Logistic regression
    c. Multiple linear regression, also called multivariate regression

Simple regression is used when there is one response or outcome variable also called *dependent variable* and one *independent* or predictor or explanatory variable. Regression is about predicting the value of [x] when you know the value of [y]. We shall have to develop the regression equation for a given dataset.

Logistic regression is used for qualitative data and is used less commonly compared to linear regression.

Likewise, multiple regression analysis is used when there is one dependent variable and two or more independent variables.

Properties of regression

    a. Regression can predict a dependent variable, the one under measurement from an independent variable.

    b. A regression model developed is used to "fit" the given dataset. A scatter plot and a line running through, is used to do the same. It is used to find the line that fits the data best.

    c. Slope parameter of *independent* variable has any difference regards to the slope parameter of dependent variable. If the difference is zero, then null hypothesis is accepted else alternative hypothesis gets accepted. This has to be a pre-specified level of significance, e.g. 0.05 if the alpha level has been chosen to be this. If an alternative hypothesis is accepted then it is concluded that there is a statistically significant association between the dependent variable and the independent variable. In that case, the model may be used to make predictions of the dependent variable.

    d. Slope parameters can be used to know the average change in dependent variable vis-à-vis change in independent variable.

Factor Analysis

If there are too many variables, then correlation regression may not be sufficient or feasible. Factor analysis may work to find the pattern of relationship among variables. It seeks to explore if the observed variables can be explained due to the presence of smaller variables called factors. Sometimes, the factor analysis is also called data analysis tool. This helps in knowing about the underlying factors and the screening of potential factors. It could do summary of variables, sampling and clustering to reduce the number of variables and retain the most important ones (Table 19.14). In particular, factor analysis can be used to explore the data for patterns, confirm our hypotheses, or reduce the many variables to a more manageable number.

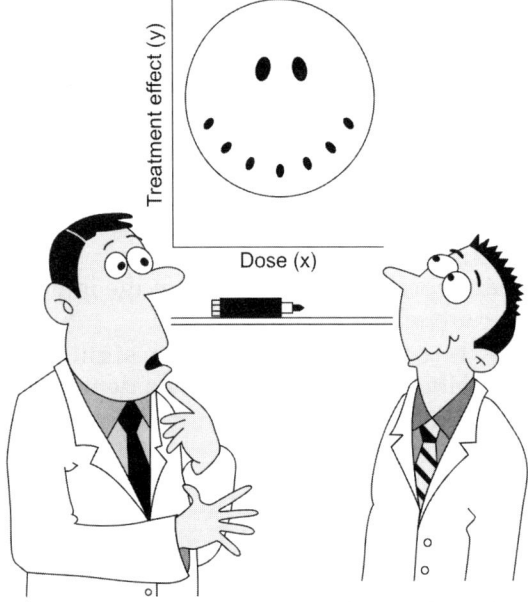

Fig. 19.11: Every relationship is not linear relationship

Table 19.14: Factor analysis questions

- How many different factors will explain pattern of relationship?
- What is the nature of those factors?
- Do hypothesized factors explain the observed data?
- How much random of unique variance does each variable has?

Properties of factor analysis

a. Factor analysis is based upon correlation analysis. Multiple, interrelated variables may be fused into smaller variables with broader dimensions.

b. Factor analysis is used to explore the nature of independent variables explaining variances in the dependent variables. This goes without saying that independent variables are not measured directly. Results of factor analysis may be tentative due to this.

Thus answers obtained by factor analysis are necessarily more hypothetical and tentative than is true when independent variables are observed directly. The inferred independent variables are called *factors*. A typical factor analysis suggests answers to four .... some .... major .... questions:

1. What is the nature of those factors?
2. How well do the hypothesized factors explain the observed data? How much purely random or unique variance does each observed variable include?

Bibliography

1. Dhikav Sethi M, Singhal A, Anand KS. Use of Potentially inappropriate Medications among patients with mild cognitive impairment and dementia. As *J Pharm and Clin Research* 2014; 7 (2): 218–220.

2. Dhikav V. Basic and Clinical Epidemiology. 1st Edition 2014; AITBS publishers, New Delhi, pp. 1–25.

3. Dhikav V. Textbook of Clinical Research. 1st Edition 2016; AITBS publishers, New Delhi, pp. 2–35.

4. Factor Analysis Downloaded from: http://ocw. jhsph. edu/courses/statisticspsychosocialresearch/pdfs/lecture8.pdf (Accessed online: 10th May, 2014).

5. Indrayan A. Medical Research. Elementary Biostatistics. AITBS Publishers, 2011; 2nd edition, pp. 27–33.

6. Interpretation of correlation coefficient. Downloaded from: http://sites.stat.psu.edu (Accessed online: 10th May, 2014).

Level of Significance

Learning objectives

The *p-value* or the probability value is the probability of obtaining a result that is equal or more extreme than the value observed in the study. In a hypothesis testing, *p-value* helps determining the significance of the results.

Null hypothesis is the hypothesis of no difference and generally in medical researching accepting it means there is no statistically significant. Accepting alternative hypothesis means, there is a statistically significant difference between the groups.

Level of Significance (*p-value*)

This is among the most common expressions used in statistics. Level of significance (*p-value*) or the *p-value* or probability value is the probability of obtaining a result "equal or more extreme" values compared to what as actually observed when the null hypothesis was true (Fig. 20.1).

In other words, its probability of committing an error when there was no difference among the groups and we end up concluding a significant difference. Probability value or simply called *p-value* is widely used in statistical hypothesis testing.

Null Hypothesis (Hypothesis of no Difference)

It is important to understand null hypothesis before understanding the *p-value*. In every experiment, there is an effect or the difference that we try to test. There may not be an effect or the difference among the groups and this lack of difference is called the null hypothesis. This is the position of devil's advocate when evaluating the result of an

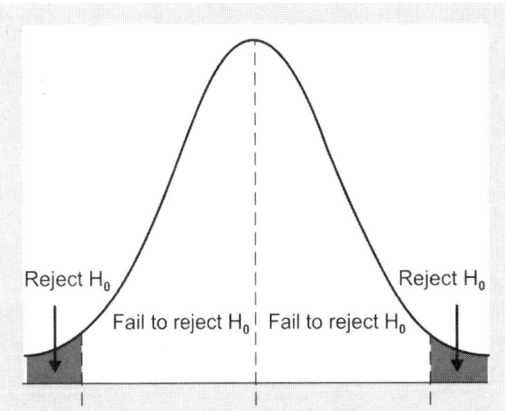 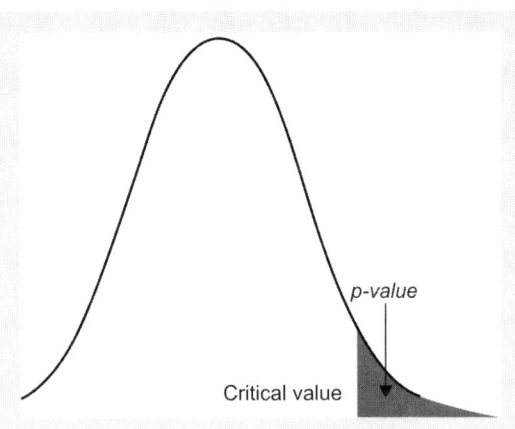

Fig. 20.1: The *p-value* is the probability of accepting or rejecting a null hypothesis and is selected before hypothesis testing begins. If the data point lies outside (i.e. the observed *p-value* is below the stated one), then the null hypothesis can be rejected. The probability of finding the statistic of interest lies in the critical zone

experiment. If the null hypothesis is true, then is no difference between the groups. The possibility of a random sampling errors should be taken into account in case if we were to label it as a "hypothesis of no difference" being true.

Testing Hypothesis

Given the collected data, is there evidence against a specified hypothesis about the corresponding parameter? Can the hypothesis be accepted or it has to be rejected. In other words, are the data consistent or not with a specified hypothesis. Hence, the significance testing is also called "hypothesis testing".

Outlines of Procedure of Hypothesis Testing

One has to start by stating hypotheses H_0 and H_a (null and alternative). One can then calculate the test statistic. This has to be followed by converting the test statistic to *p-value* and interpret the same based upon the pre-set alpha levels. Thus, before doing any work with the data, we must decide on a tolerance level. That means, how low must be our *p-value* be before we reject the null hypothesis? The significance level or the α hence must be decided before studying the data!

In simple words, the *p-value* evaluates how well the sample data supports the argument if the null hypothesis was true or not. It measures how compatible is the data with the null hypothesis. In general, if *p-value* is higher than the stated alpha level; null hypothesis is true, else it is untrue. A lower than stated alpha level (*p-value*) is a good ground to reject the null hypothesis (Fig. 20.2).

Probability values or the *p-values* started around a century back and have been criticized and misused too. So we should not be obsessed with *p-value* as such and there is more to statistics than just *p-value*. It should be used along with the alpha level to increase the confidence of scientific community in the research.

Indeed when Sir Fisher introduced *p-values*, he never intended such values to be the sole deciding factor for study validity. As per Fisher it was a part of the process that incorporated scientific reasoning, experimentation, analysis and scientific conclusions. As per Fisher, a scientific fact produced as a result of a properly designed experiment will always yield a significant *p-value*. However, it may need repeated studies for confirmation. Beginners may take *p-value* for granted without going into the depth of hypothesis, which could be misleading.

Guidelines for p-Values

There may be an untold pressure among students to find a low *p-values* which are significant and there may be misunderstanding among them to correctly use the *p-value*.

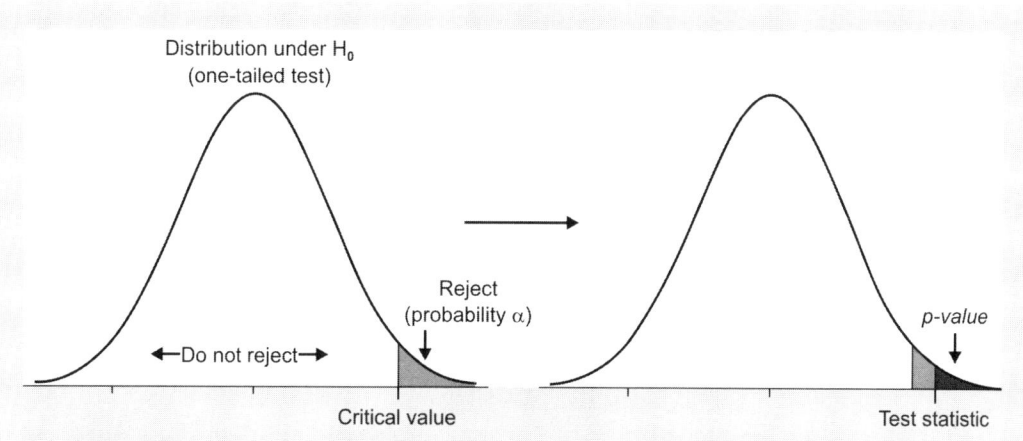

Fig. 20.2: Acceptance or rejection of null hypothesis depends upon pre-stated *p-value*

Following are useful guidelines

a. *Do not just mention the stated p-value*: Rather than saying *p-value* < 0.05 or > 0.05; one should give the exact *p-value*.

b. *Make it comprehensive*: While discussing *p-values*, one should include both positive and negative studies as to give a balanced look.

c. *Effect size does matter*: One should keep in mind that *p-value* represents the finding that the difference between two groups is statistically significant or not; so we should look at the fact as to what effect size does the *p-value* is mentioning about. Also, one should note as to what is the relevance of the same.

d. *Think of alternative hypothesis*: We should focus on the alternative hypothesis too rather than just rejecting the null. One should ask him selves/her selves as to what is the relevance of accepting the alternative hypothesis.

Bibliography

1. Correctly interpret *p-value*. http://blog.minitab.com/blog/adventures-in-statistics-2/how-to-correctly-interpret-p-values (Downloaded on February 9th 2017).

2. *P-values*. http://www.statsdirect.com/help/basics/p_values.htm (Downloaded on February 9th 2017).

3. Why do we compare *p-value* to significance level in hypothesis testing of mean? http://stats.stackexchange.com/questions/124178/why-do-we-compare-p-value-to-significance-level-in-hypothesis-testing-of-mean (Downloaded on February 9th 2017).

Relative Risk and Odds Ratio

Learning objectives

Odds ratio is the Odds of having diseases among exposed divided by the Odds of disease among the unexposed. If the relative risk is 1, then the association of exposure with the disease is unlikely but if it more than one then the risk of disease among exposed is high. Odds ratio and relative risks are often confused. Both measure association between a binary outcome variable and a predictor variable. Odds ratio is the ratio of two Odds whereas the relative risk is the ratio of two probabilities (hence called risk ratio).

Introduction

Relative Risk (RR) or the Risk Ratio is the probability of an outcome occurring in an exposed group compared to those who are unexposed. For example, one can compare the frequency of cough among those who are exposed to pollution compared to those who are unexposed.

Odds Ratio (OR) is a measure of association between exposure and outcome. OR represents the Odds that an outcome will occur with a exposure compared to without exposure.

Ratio is the number (a) of observations in a given group with a given characteristic divided by the number (b) of observations without the given characteristic. Odds is the probability of finding the outcome of interest. Mathematically, the probability that an event will occur divided by the probability that the event will not occur = p/1–p.

Odds ratio is Odds that a patient is exposed to the risk factor divided by the Odds that a control is exposed. This is calculated using case control ratio.

Odds ratio can be calculated in a cohort study and in a case-control study. The exposure Odds ratio is equal to the disease Odds ratio. Relative risk can only be calculated in a cohort study. Odds ratio can be a measure of relative risk in case control study.

Interpreting Odds ratio		
Value of OR	*Interpretation*	*Conclusion*
1.0	Odds of exposure in cases and controls is same	Exposure is not associated with disease
> 1.0	Odds are higher in cases	Exposure is risk factor
< 1.0	Odds in controls higher	Exposure is protective

Case-Control Study

In a *case-control* study, we do not know the incidence in the exposed population or the incidence in the nonexposed population because we start with diseased people (cases) and nondiseased people (controls). Hence, in a case-control study we *cannot* calculate the relative risk directly. Another measure of association, the *Odds ratio,* can be obtained from a case-control study. The *Odds ratio* can be used instead of the relative risk in a case control study; while the latter is used more commonly in cohort study. That means, even though we cannot calculate a relative risk from a case-control study, under many conditions, we can obtain a very good *estimate* of the relative risk from a case-control study using the Odds ratio.

For example, in a study of vascular risk factors in patients with dementias; when we start with cases (dementia), and controls (healthy), we do not know the incidence of vascular risk factors in cases and controls; hence we will compare Odds of diabetes and hypertension (vascular risks) in both cases and controls. This is because both exposure and the disease have occurred before the start of the study.

Cohort Study

In a cohort study, the Odds ratio is defined as the *ratio of the Odds of development of disease in exposed persons to the Odds of development of disease in nonexposed persons.* In a *case-control study,* we cannot calculate the relative risk directly to determine whether there is an association between the exposure and the disease. This is because, having started with cases and controls rather than with exposed and nonexposed persons, we do not have information about the incidence of disease in exposed versus nonexposed persons. However, we can use the Odds ratio as a measure of the association between exposure and disease in a case-control study. But we ask different questions: "What are the Odds that a case was exposed?"

Cohort studies use the incidences to assess the risk and compare the incidence in the exposed (incidence$_1$) to the incidences in the nonexposed (incidence$_0$) and hence calculate the risk ratio (ϕ)

$$\phi = \frac{\text{Incidence}_1}{\text{Incidence}_0}$$

The main disadvantage of cohort is the long induction between exposure and disease may cause delays. This design is suitable for the study of rare diseases and require large sample sizes to accrue sufficient numbers. When studying many people information can be limited in scope and accuracy hence data entry should be meticulously done. Case-control studies were developed to help overcome some of these limitations.

After having studied both Odds ratio and relative risk, it is important to know the difference between the two. This is important

as to untrained eye, the may look to be all the same. It is important to know that both measure association between a binary outcome variable and a continuous or binary predictor variable. The names are sometimes used interchangeably. They should not be because they are actually interpreted differently. So it is important to keep them separate and to be precise in the language you use. The general rule though is that if the prevalence of the disease is < 10% or so, the relative risk and the Odds ratio will be approximately the same. The rarer the disease, the closer is the likely approximation between Odds ratio and relative risk. If it is statistically sound to do so, Odds ratio is generally safer, easier and less open to misinterpretation.

Absolute Risk

Absolute risk is the risk of developing a disease over a time period. All humans have risk of developing diseases like diabetes, heart disease, cancer stroke. For example, if risk of developing diabetes is 10%, then the AR is 10% or 0.1.

Absolute risk involves people who contract disease due to an exposure and it does not consider those who are sick but have not been exposed. This is the number of people experiencing an event (good or bad) in relation to the population at risk.

In a cardiology clinic with an outpatient attendance of 100 and a total of 20 patients had diabetes; what is the absolute risk? 20/100 = 0.2 or 20%. Likewise, in a gynecology clinic with an attendance of 150; a total of 30 women had polycystic ovaries. What is the AR? 30/150 = 0.2 or 20%.

Absolute Risk Reduction (ARR)

Risk means probability of developing disease/ and or outcome.

Absolute risk reduction or ARR is the size difference between two treatments. It tells how much is one treatment better compared to the other in reducing the number of people who experience a given outcome compared to the other. That means, as a result of treatment is the risk of an event reduced significantly or not.

ARR is basically risk difference between control and the treated group.

ARR is easy to calculate and gives an easy idea about the benefit of treatment.

For example, in a clinical trial of migraine where a preventive treatment is being explored only 2 out of 100 people experience migraine compared to 4 out of 100; the risk difference is 2%. So 50% fewer people get migraine if they are on anti-migraine drugs.

Relative Risk Reduction (RRR)

Relative risk reducing or RRR tells us as to how much did the treatment reduce the bad outcomes in the intervention group compared to the control group.

In the previous example of migraine prevention the absolute risk reduction is just 2% but the relative risk reduction is 50% which sounds more impressive! Cost of treatment and side effects determine other things.

Number Needed to Treat

Another way to express risk reduction is Number Needed to Treat (NNT). This is inverse of absolute risk reduction. Suppose if a drug reduces the bad event outcome from 50 to 40% the ARR is 10% (0.1) and the NNT will be 1/ARR = 0.1 = 10 (Table 21.1).

Relative Risk

Relative Risk (RR) compares the risks in two different groups of people, e.g. smokers and nonsmokers or those who are exposed to pollution as opposed to those who are not.

Relative risk is a measure of the strength of association based on prospective studies (cohort studies) in cohort studies like Odds ratio in case control studies.

RR is nothing but the ratio of incidence of disease in exposed individuals to the incidence of disease in nonexposed individuals and is calculated from a cohort/prospective studies (Table 21.2).

  i. If RR > 1, there is a positive association

  ii. If RR < 1, there is a negative association

Relative risk is calculated as:
RR = Risk in exposed/risk in nonexposed.

Table 21.2: Interpretation of relative risk

RR	Interpretation
RR = 1	Risk in exposed and unexposed is equal and there is no association
RR > 1	Risk in exposed is greater than non-exposed and this is a positive association; could possibly be causal
RR < 1	Risk in exposed is less than nonexposed and this is a negative association; could possibly be protective

Table 21.1: Advantages and disadvantages of number needed to treat analysis

Advantages	Disadvantages
• Summarize results of a clinical trial or for decision-making	• Cannot be used for meta-analysis
• Better than relative risk or relative risk reduction or Odds ratio	• Risk benefits cannot be calculated for an individual patient
• Expression of risk is simple	• It entails the number of individuals that need to be treated rather than the size of the benefit

In a cohort of 3000 patients exposed to the air pollution in Delhi, a total of 84 patients developed chronic bronchitis in a follow-up period of 3 years 2014 to 2016 while out of a total population followed up from Shimla, only 28 patients developed chronic bronchitis. What is the relative risk?

• Incidence among exposed = 84/3000 = 28/1000
• Incidence among nonexposed = 50/5000 = 10/1000
• RR = Risk in exposed/risk in nonexposed.

Relative risk = 28/10 = 2.8; a RR > 1 means it is a positive association implying that being in air pollution is a risk factor for chronic bronchitis.

It is important to know that we cannot derive incidence from case-control studies as they begin with diseased people (cases) and nondiseased people (controls), therefore, cannot calculate relative risk directly but, we can use another method called an Odds ratio.

	Develop disease	Do not develop disease
Exposed	a	b
Not exposed	c	d

Odds Ratio (OR)

As stated elsewhere; in a *case-control* study, we do not know the incidence in the exposed population or the incidence in the nonexposed population because we start with diseased people (cases) and nondiseased people (controls); hence, in a case-control study we *cannot* calculate the relative risk directly as is done in prospective cohorts. The *Odds ratio,* can be obtained from either a cohort or a case-control study; more so in the latter. Even though we cannot calculate a relative risk from a case-control study, under many conditions, we can obtain a very good *estimate* of the relative risk from a case-control study using the Odds ratio. In case-control studies, we discuss the *proportion* of the cases who were exposed and the *proportion* of the controls who were exposed and compare both, i.e. = Odds that an exposed individual develops disease/Odds that a nonexposed individual develops disease

$$= ab/cd$$

When does OR becomes RR

a. Odds ratio becomes an estimate of relative risk when cases are representative of diseased population.

b. When controls are representative of population without disease.

c. When the disease being studied occurs at low frequency.

Confidence Interval

Confidence interval aims to give an idea about how confident one is about the study estimates; especially of the treatment effects. This is very important in clinical trials. Even when a study has an implacable quality, the stated results could occur due to chance. In statistics; there is a method of dealing with such an uncertainty that tells as to what extent we are confident about the estimates of the study. This is called Confidence Interval (CI). If the confidence interval is narrow; one can be more confident about the findings being the "real difference" rather than due to chance alone. This is usually expressed as 95% confidence interval or commonly abbreviated as 95% CI. This actually represents the range about which we are 95% confident of finding the variable of interest.

Bibliography

1. Andrade C. Understanding relative risk, Odds ratio, and related terms: as simple as it can get. *J Clin Psychiatry*. 2015 Jul;76(7):e857–61. doi: 10.4088/JCP.15f10150.

2. Relative risk and Odds ratio. http://www.mdedge.com/jfponline/article/65515/relative-risks-and-Odds-ratios-whats-difference (Downloaded on February 9th 2017).

3. The difference between relative risk and Odds ratio. http://www.theanalysisfactor.com/the-difference-between-relative-risk-and-Odds-ratios/(Downloaded on February 9th 2017).

Thesis Writing

Learning objectives

A thesis is a statement of the scientific work that has focused on the ideas and the work one has generated typically for a university degree. Thesis should make clear statements, and should be neatly written and well organized. The most important thing is to stay focused while describing a thesis.

WHAT IS A THESIS?

An online dictionary defines thesis as Thesis (noun)—a "proposition maintained by argument" or in other worlds, "a dissertation advancing original research".

WHY IS IT IMPORTANT TO WRITE THESIS?

It is important to know that normally PG students only have to write one thesis (unless someone does PhD after MSc/MD). At the end, one can add "Dr" to his/her name. So a doctoral thesis is valuable.

Takes Lot of Efforts

Writing a thesis is hard, and painstaking work. One may have already done the fun part (the research); but the writing may be quite a bit of an effort. It is unlike any other document and thesis writing is not a marketable skill! That means, it cannot easily be learnt. It is a painstaking process that takes a lot of time too.

WHO READS THESIS?

Apart from the guide, it will be read by thesis committee; also called doctoral committee. Of course it goes for evaluation to at least two different experts as well. A thesis is therefore a sacrosanct academic document and needs to be prepared sincerely.

MSc/MD Thesis

Purpose of postgraduate thesis is a good training of research methods, biostatistics and be able to form hypothesis and work under guidance. The student should demonstrate analytical skills about a topic that has been given to him/her. It should be noted that it is not the end of the research work but first significant part of the academic work that the candidate has done.

PhD Thesis

This is the highest form of thesis. It may open a new area and provides unifying framework. It may resolve the long-standing questions and thoroughly explores scientific areas. It may also contradict the existing knowledge or experimentally validate a theory. It may have several additional features (Table 22.1).

Table 22.1: Features of PhD thesis

- Provides empirical data
- Derives superior algorithms
- Develops new methodology
- Develops new tool
- Produces negative result

Getting Started
Title

This is the front page and it should have the title mentioned.

Certificate

This goes like this: This is to certify that the work embodied in this thesis entitled, "..........................." is original and has been carried out by .... under the supervision of .... The work has not been submitted in part or in full, for any other degree or diploma for this or any other university.

This has to be signed by the research scholar, guide and the dean who will forward the work to the university.

Declaration

This is signed by the research candidate.

This is to certify that the work embodied in this thesis entitled, "..............." is original and free from any form of falsification, fabrication and plagiarism. I shall be solely responsible for any such dispute arising out of my doctoral work.

Dedication

This is usually in name of someone whom the author feels; could be family member, guide or anyone else.

Acknowledgments

This is a very important page, where we acknowledge all those who have helped us in carrying out this work. It normally starts with thanking the guide under whom the work has been done and ends by thanking the almighty. It should be positive, balanced and should not contain unnecessary flattery.

List of abbreviations

This entails the use of terms that are frequent in the thesis.

Table of contents

A brief template of table of contents is give below. This should be developed right in beginning to make things easier. It may consist of the following:

Abstract

This is a widely read part of the thesis. This lies right in the beginning and should be comprehensive. This part attracts first attention of the reviewer hence should be error free. One should do a quick spell check before considering it a final copy. It should be professionally written; preferably in a manner as to be able to send the manuscript in an international journal, i.e. background, introduction, material and methods, results, discussion, conclusion, etc. It should represent a snapshot of the whole study and should be a standalone feature.

Introduction

After the abstract, this is most likely read part. The problem proposed to be studied is introduced in this section. It should help the reader to acquaint with the topic. This should not be very detailed; may be 2–3 pages to 5–7 pages. One should be brief in introduction yet at the same time, cover what was known about this topic and why was it chosen. Also, what were the knowledge gap and how could this work contribute to the advancement of knowledge should be highlighted.

Review of literature

This should be as detailed as possible. This should reflect state-of-art of the knowledge and be properly referenced. One common mistake many students make is to cut and paste the review of literature. Remember in all good universities; the theses are checked for piracy. It is critical that we do not cut and paste here.

This section reflects extensive review of literature done by the investigator. In this section what is already known about the topic is written including the lacunae. Just quoting the literature verbatim will not serve the purpose. It is important to make it coherent, relevant and easily readable knowledge. It helps the investigator to gain good knowledge in that field of inquiry. It also helps the investigator to have insight on different methodologies that could be applied.

Rationale of study

Study rationale should properly be explained as to what led to this study. This is often scrutinized as this is the basis of forming a research hypothesis.

Aim and objective

Aim is a single broad statement of intent of the study. This is a very important and pivotal section of thesis and everything else in the study is centered around it. The aim and objectives of the proposed study should be stated very clearly. The objective stated should be specific, achievable and measurable and too many objectives to be avoided. Even just one clearly stated relevant objective for a study would be good enough. If there is more than one objective the objectives can be presented in the appropriate order of importance. The following is a rough guide as to how to write index of a thesis.

Serial number	Contents list of abbreviations
Chapter 1	Abstract
Chapter 2	Introduction
Chapter 3	Review of literature
Chapter 4	Rationale of study
Chapter 5	Aim and objectives
Chapter 6	Research question and hypothesis
Chapter 7	Material and methods
Chapter 8	Results
Chapter 9	Discussion
Chapter 10	Strengths and limitations of the study
Chapter 11	Conclusions
Chapter 12	Summary
Chapter 13	References
Chapter 14	Brief Biodata of the author
Chapter 15	Appendices
	Publications

Bibliography

1. Centre for writing studies: thesis writing tips. http://www.cws.illinois.edu/workshop/writers/tips/thesis/ (Downloaded February 9th 2017).
2. Developing a thesis. http://writingcenter.fas.harvard.edu/pages/developing-thesis (Downloaded February 9th 2017).
3. How to write PhD thesis? http://newt.phys.unsw.edu.au/~jw/thesis.html (Downloaded February 9th 2017).
4. How to write thesis? http://www.ldeo.columbia.edu/~martins/sen_sem/thesis_org.html (Downloaded February 9th 2017).
5. Skills needed for writing a thesis. https://www.skillsyouneed.com/learn/dissertation-writing.html (Downloaded February 9th 2017).
6. Thesis writing guidelines. https://educationguide.tue.nl/programs/graduate-school/masters-programs/computer-science-and-engineering/graduation/thesis-writing-guidelines/ (Downloaded February 9th 2017).

Getting Published

Learning objectives

Publication is the essence of science something that scientists live everyday. In general, there is a general saying, "perform or perish" and it has been replaced in science by "publish or perish". There is a genuine pressure that we feel on the people to publish. This tendency is increasing in India day by day. Majority of Indian medical institutions engage in medical research now and some of them are very productive. So learning how to publish is very important.

Introduction

Often new students find it dauntingly hard to think of manuscripts. When randomly surveyed, Indian medical graduates trying to get hold of thesis topics will seem to be lost during their MD curriculum; that is because, they have no previous background in research. All of sudden they enter into unknown territory. Therefore, in the beginning guidance, clear directions and assistance is needed.

Select a Topic

Selecting a topic is difficult, because several thoughts come to mind. However, something that you have connected with right from beginning will help. For example, in pharmacology if you liked calcium channel blockers, or arrhythmias in medicine or hernia in surgery or premenstrual tension in gynecology could be your broad thesis/manuscript papers. Often professors in India would like to start you with case reports or case series. If you get to write an original article early on in your career, you could be lucky.

Literature Search

Once you get an idea of the broad area; think of literature search. This will give you a better idea as to what others have done and what has been produced earlier. It may take lot of time.

Look into www.pubmed.com or www. google.com or www.googlescholar.com. Be aware if you are a China/Russia passed medical student; then Google related applications do not work in general in China or Russia. They work nicely in India though. Look at full length articles if you interested in that topic seriously (Fig. 23.1). Abstract contain only the concise information and are not enough!

Title/Aim

If you writing a manuscript, select a short and informative title. It should be eye-catching one

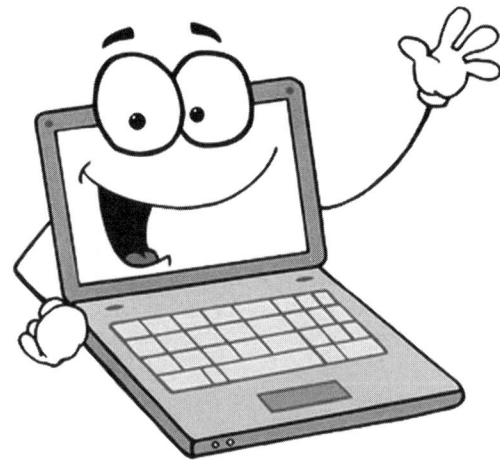

Fig. 23.1: Searching literature is an art and science and using appropriate keywords can yield useful information in shortest possible time

that gets the reader's attention! Short titles rather than long and explanatory are better. Keep the reader guessing rather than explaining everything in title itself.

Aim vs Objective

Aim is the ultimate outcome that are seeking and the objective the way and means by which we shall achieve the same. Objectives can be many, but aim has to be one. Objectives can be primary and secondary. For the sake of simplicity; one should keep the objectives to minimum number. Sometimes when we become enthusiastic we may keep many of them but keeping them to 1–2 is better (Fig. 23.2).

Hypothesis

This is the backbone of your research and it should be thoughtfully crafted. Be prepared with null and alternative hypothesis. All major journals will look into this with *Google eyes*. They would want to know if you had formulated it correctly and if the results and discussion which has been presented actually match-up to the same.

Research Question

This is an extension of your hypothesis and is it actually something that you are investigating and trying to find the answer of. A research question is the workable hypothesis that you are trying to find the answer of!

Material and Methods

This is the most valuable part of the paper which is read by serious readers. Indeed if they have been described nicely, then the results are going to be read as well (Fig. 23.3).

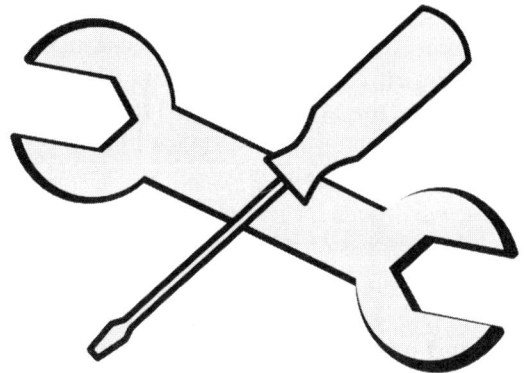

Fig. 23.3: Working on a manuscript involves carefully engineered steps

Else, most readers would stop here! Be descriptive, and express, "how can someone else do the same by reading the section you are describing". That means, it should be the "workable material and methods".

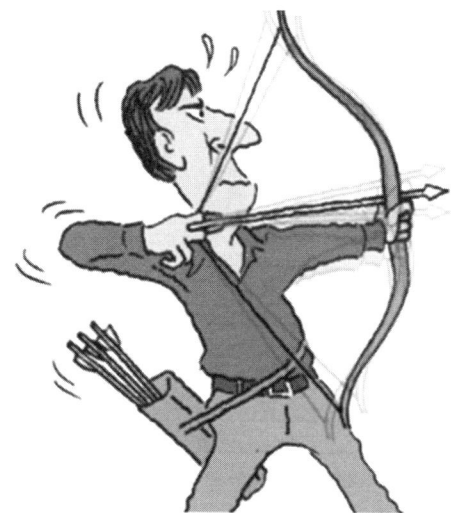
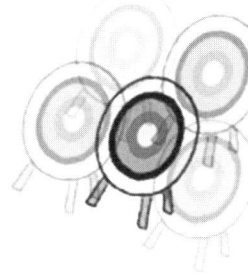

Fig. 23.2: Students often get confused between aim and objectives

Some journals want the same under following heads:

a. *Population*: What is the total number you have studied? How did you select the population? How did you decide that this was a representative sample size? Was it a hospital based study or a community sample?

b. *Sample size*: Very important determinant of the study. It can be small or large. Was it a convenient sampling or was it something you selected based upon a formula? Was statistician consulted before the study began? How did you select alpha level (alpha) or beta level or power of the study?

c. *Consent* was informed consent taken and the process of taking the consent.

d. *Ethical approval*: Nowadays, it is important to take ethical approvals of the projects and one should have be explicit in this regard. In India, there is a clinical trial registry and it is important to the trial registered here before considering publications.

e. *Timelines*: If we were to submit a project, then the clear timelines will have to be submitted to funding agency.

f. *Budgets and audits*: Projects sponsored by pharma companies, will have to be submitted in detail and manpower, instruments, investigator fees, site charges, etc. will have to be explained in detail. Process of auditing will have to be clear.

Discussion

This is most widely read part of paper where the researcher actually describes the same in detail. The results of the study are compared with the studies that have been done earlier. This will give the readers and idea as to how would your results be different from others.

Conclusion

This is an important part and should be kept short. One could describe the key findings and highlight the need for further research.

Sending the Article to a Journal

Your guide will push you if you were doing MSc/MD/PhD/DM thesis and were trying to publish a paper to send your article in a good journal. Peer reviewed journals are good journals, especially the ones run by societies. Select one of those for you!

Most journals have online submissions nowadays and the websites are friendly. You just need to browse through the sites so that you can submit by being there and follow the instructions. There are options of going back and change something. So submission is an easy process. Make sure you have informed all your authors and your guides when you submitting a manuscript. All authors listen will get a submission email.

Peer Review

Most journals have this process where the journal article is sent for blind review. This is a simple process, where the experienced authors who have written manuscript earlier are made 'judges' and give blind comments on the manuscripts they have been sent. The comments sent by the reviewers are blind and detailed.

They will have to be answered one by one. Please do not be intimated by extensive nature of comments and feel that your paper would be rejected. Even when comments are detailed and answered properly, the paper gets accepted! Eventually!

However, one will have to persist and not to be disdained (Fig. 23.4).

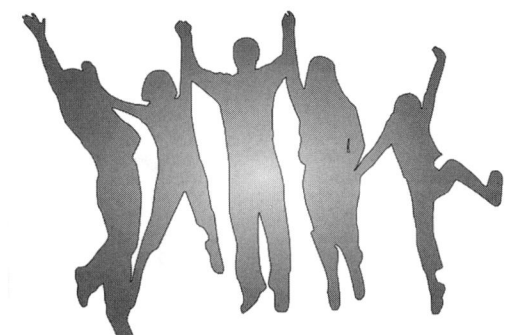

Fig. 23.4: Peer review enhances the quality of the manuscript

Answering Queries of Peer Reviewers

Peer review is a rigorous process and can be demotivating for the new scientists; for the seasoned scientists, it is a usual process that they sill through easily. One should answer the reviewers point by point and one has to be very objective about the same. One should preferably substantiate the same using some references. Even till last minute, reviewers and editors might want some corrections. Do not be discouraged by the same. Try to adhere to guidelines.

Getting Published

Normally, you are sent a proof of the paper before publishing. Even good journals can have error in manuscript; especially in titles, your names, addresses, affiliations, etc. so check the manuscript thoroughly before approving it for publication finally (Fig. 23.5). Sometimes gross errors may be there and detected just at last minute!

Several websites track the progress of researchers nowadays. One could make an account on one of these. These could calculate the h-index, i-10 index and number of citations in 5 years and also the impact points (research gate). In other words, your progress gets monitored automatically.

Deciding Authorship

An author is the person who has made substantial contribution to the paper. Generally,

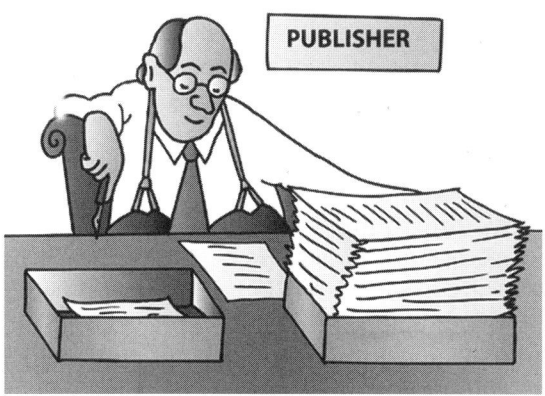

Fig. 23.5: Getting linked with Google scholar/ Research gate is important as it gives a wider reach to the published work

this is the person who has been involved at almost stages of the paper, i.e. inception, hypothesis, collecting information, executing study, collecting data and writing the report. Nowadays, it is not uncommon to see someone getting involved at a later stage. That means, someone could still come in at the editorial stage if the language of the paper needs major overhauling. Likewise, a statistician too can come at a later stages if the paper is unclear about the statistical methods used.

International Committee of Medical Editors defines the author as following:

a. Involved from the conception and design of the manuscript.
b. Participated in interpretation of research findings.
c. Drafting of the article of revising the paper by providing the critical inputs needed for publication.
d. Final approval of the paper for publication.
e. Data collection alone, funding, general supervision does not alone qualify for the authorship.

"Gifted Authorship"

This is something that Indian authors are often confronted with. Whenever, a new manuscript is being prepared, there will always be some people around who would like to be the part of the same. One should however avoid the temptation of involving people in the same. In authors experience, the 'gifted authors' mostly do not value the manuscript and at some point or others will lead to problematic outcome.

Research Credits

Nowadays, it is common in Indian medical institutions to have publications as the basis of promotions. Slowly, it seems the "time bound" promotions will get replaced by a better system of 'credit based' promotions where publications will come at forefront. Researchers get a score and based upon the same the researchers get promoted to medical and biomedical institutions around the world.

Copyright

It is not uncommon to see at junior level specially to have infringement of copyright laws. Keep in mind, that if you copy someone else's work and make it look 'your own', it is unethical!

Be aware that this is a substandard practice and is never going to make you better researcher. Following should be kept in mind:

a. Cite the original author whenever, some material has been taken from his/her article.

b. Take due permission from author/publisher or both when you are going to reproduce the work done by someone.

c. Before modifying some figure or flow-chart, take permission from the authors.

d. Do not copy and cite in the reference list or provide acknowledgment.

Plagiarism

This is an important issue in today's world with a large number of people interested in publications. There is a tremendous amount of race going on and hence, it is not uncommon to see people copying each other's work to get recognition. Plagiarism is simply copying the other's work to get recognition. It is therefore, important not to copy and write your own stuff! Plagiarism detecting software have now come and are able to identify if the manuscripts have been copied or not. Plagiarism is a major ethical offence!

Nowadays a very tough standard regarding plagiarism is the "five (consecutive) word" rule, which holds that, if there are five consecutive words identical to someone else's writing, then one would be held guilty of plagiarism.

Conflict of Interest

One has to declare if someone has some conflict of interest as to if someone accepted some favors from some company to write in their favors or modified the manuscript as per requirement. Though uncommon, but still one should declare this while writing a manuscript to a journal. It is generally expressed as:

Conflict of interest: None

This will save the scientist or medical doctor from participating in a manuscript whose results may be clouded.

Duplicate Publications

Someone may submit the paper to more than one journal and this is counted as a duplicate publication. One must not do this. In modern world, a journal will always ask if this paper has been published somewhere or is being considered somewhere for publication. This is another major ethical offence to have two papers which are identical!

Communicating to Press

Media in modern India is independent and proactive. They often reach out to the people in scientific world and ask them if anything new has happened. It is a common temptation to discuss things at length with people who are in press. However, if there is a finding that has been published in the peer review journal and has been well-documented should be communicated to the press. While such a communication is being done, care should be taken to do so in laymen language so that everyone can understand. Technical details should be avoided. Same goes true when a scientist or a medical doctor appears on TV or Radio shows.

Scientific Frauds

This is a rare event when a scientist or a medical doctor fabricates the results of the studies done by someone and then publishes the same under his or her name! This is a gross scientific misconduct. In some nations, for this behavior, even the name of the doctor can be struck from medical register records.

In India, such issues are slowly getting addressed. Now the medical editors active seek the articles that are original and check their originality. Moreover, most journals in Indian subcontinent will ask the contributors to submit a certificate that the work done is original and has not been copied. Likewise, it is also needed that an undertaking is given by the researchers that the workdone has neither been not submitted nor been published anywhere.

Editorial Responsibilities

Editors have a major responsibility in ensuring the reliability of the contents that they publish. It is prime concern of the biomedical editor that the material to be published has all the accurate, reliable, non-plagiarised contents. Additionally, they have to check for plagiarism as well. They have to ensure that the content that has been submitted to them is 'ethical' and has been scrutinized by the institutional ethical committees as well.

In India, in particular, nowadays, this is a growing challenge to be able to scrutinize manuscripts that come to the editors for publication. It is a full time job to ensure accuracy, check plagiarism and follow the individual ones to the logical conclusion.

Bibliography

1. International committee of medical journal editors: defining role of authors and contributors. http:// www.icmje.org/recommendations/ browse/roles-and-responsibilities/defining-the-role-of-authors-and-contributors.html (Downloaded February 9th 2017).

2. Learn how to publish papers. https://www. coursera.org/learn/how-to-write-a-scientific-paper (Downloaded February 9th 2017).

3. Learning publications. https://www. globalreporting.org/services/preparation/ Publications/learning publications/Pages/ default.aspx (Downloaded February 9th 2017).

4. Publication guidelines. http://publicationethics. org/resources/guidelines (Downloaded February 9th 2017).

5. Research to publication. http://rtop.bmj.com/ (Downloaded February 9th 2017).

Plagiarism, Falsification, Fabrication in Medical Research

WHAT IS PLAGIARISM?

Plagiarism is the act of stealing someone else's work and attempting to "pass it off" as your own (Fig. 24.1). This can apply to anything, from papers to photographs to songs, even ideas!

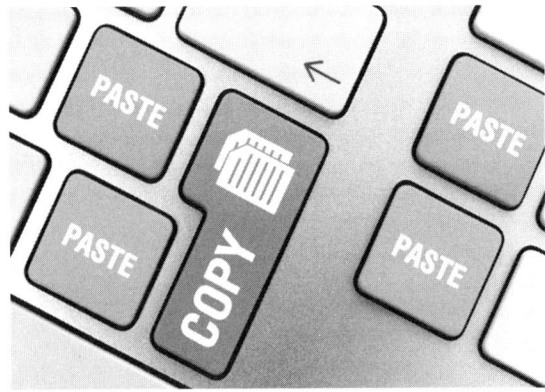

Fig. 24.1: Plagiarism is to steal and pass off the ideas or words of another as one's own. This cut and paste practice is rampant and is a cause for concern in the publication world

Plagiarism is the act of presenting the words, ideas, images, sounds, or the creative expression of others as your own.

Research Misconduct

Research misconduct is defined as *fabrication, falsification,* or *plagiarism* in *proposing, performing,* or *reviewing research,* or in *reporting research results* (*US Office of Science and Technology Policy*). The following are the commonly used terms:

- *Fabrication* is the description of experiments not actually performed, the invention of

data not actually collected, and/or the reporting of these experiments and results.

- *Falsification* is manipulating research materials, equipment, or processes, or changing or omitting data or results such that the research is not accurately represented in the research record.

- *Cooking* is retaining and reporting only the data that fits the theory and discarding others.

- *Trimming* is the smoothing of irregularities to make the data look more accurate and precise than they really are.

Copyright

This is a commonly used term came across while searching the literature. Copyright is "a form of protection provided by the laws" to the authors of 'original works of authorship,' including literary, dramatic, musical, artistic, and certain other intellectual works. This protection is available to both published and unpublished works (Fig. 24.2).

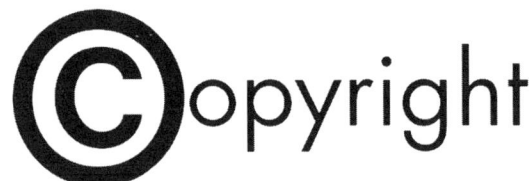

Fig. 24.2: Copyright is a legal right that is conferred upon to the creator of this idea by the laws of the land. This holds that the original creator of the work has exclusive right for its use and distribution

WHAT IS FAIR USE?

"Fair Use"" is a statute under copyright law that allows for the use of *limited portions* of a work that has copyright **without** having to have permission from the original author. It was created for the purposes of education and research. It is a little harder to pin down than plagiarism or copyright. I mean, what qualifies as a "limited portion" could be hard to define.

The copyright office rules are not very helpful on defining what a "limited portion" is. It only states that "there is no specific number of words, lines, or notes that may safely be taken without permission." When using someone else's work, it is best to always give credit where credit's due, even if using only a small part. If you are unsure, then ask for permission. Table 24.1 gives examples of fair usage.

Table 24.1: Fair use
Commentary
Search engines
Criticism
News reporting
Research

One can clearly see in Table 24.1 that "fair usage" is not specific enough.

Copying/Cut and Paste

The most well-known and, sadly, the most common type of plagiarism is the simplest: copying. If you copy someone else's work and put your name on it, you have plagiarised.

Unintentional

a. *Paraphrasing poorly*: Changing a few words without changing the sentence structure of the original, or changing the sentence structure but not the words.
b. *Quoting poorly*: Putting quotation marks around part of a quotation but not around all of it, or putting quotation marks around a passage that is partly paraphrased and partly quoted.
c. *Citing poorly*: Omitting an occasional citation or citing inaccurately.

Intentional

d. Passing off as one's own pre-written papers from the internet or other sources.
e. Copying an essay or article from the internet, online source, or electronic database without quoting or giving credit.
f. Cutting and pasting from more than one source to create a paper without quoting or giving credit.
g. Borrowing words or ideas from other students or sources without giving credit.

Patchwork Plagiarism

The second kind of plagiarism is similar to copying and is perhaps the second most common type of plagiarism: patchwork plagiarism. This occurs when the plagiariser borrows the "phrases and clauses from the original source and weaves them into his own writing" without putting the phrases in quotation marks or citing the author.

Paraphrasing

The third type of plagiarism is called para-phrasing plagiarism. This occurs when the plagiariser paraphrases or summarises another's work without citing the source. Even changing the words a little or using synonyms but retaining the author's essential thoughts, sentence structure, and/or style without citing the source is still considered plagiarism.

Plagiarism of Self

The use of previous work for a separate assignment and this is not uncommon as well. Although the work is original but using them again and again in same language is cheating as well.

Avoiding Plagiarism

Avoiding plagiarism is quite simple. The best method for avoiding it is to simply be honest; when you have used a source in your paper, give credit where it is due. Acknowledge the author of the original work you have used. In order to properly quote your sources, one should consult the style manual that would be appropriate for the research. In most cases, your professor will tell you which style would be preferred. If your professor does not indicate which manual to use, be sure to ask. Vancouver and Harvard are two commonly used referencing methods.

Following are general instructions to avoid plagiarism:

a. Use your own work as often as possible. Quoting and citing sources is usually required and inevitable when doing research—that's how you "back up" your own work. But using someone else's work excessively can be construed as plagiarism.

b. Quote and/or cite your sources properly. Develop a topic based on previously written material but write something new and original.

c. One can rely on opinions of experts on a topic but improve upon those opinions and develop your own. One should give credit to researchers while making your own contribution.

Bibliography

1. Plagiarism detector": http://www.quetext. com/(Downloaded on February 9th 2017).
2. What is fair use? http://fairuse.stanford.edu/ overview/fair-use/what-is-fair-use/ (Downloaded on February 9th 2017).
3. What is plagiarism? http://www.plagiarism. org/(Downloaded on February 9th 2017).

Taking Consent in Medical Research

Learning objectives

Consent in research setting is called "informed consent" as all the information has been passed onto the participants. Education and information exchange should take place between the researcher and the participant in an objective manner.

The information should be passed in a manner easily understood by the subjects and the local language could be used to facilitate understanding. Use of audiovisual tools can make things simple and easily reproducible as well.

Consent

Informed consent is a process which is designed to empower the individual to make a voluntary informed decision regarding participation in the research. Voluntary consent means that the participants were able to consent, were not being coerced to do the study and understood the risks and benefit involved.

It is generally said that the medical advances should not require some people to sacrifice their health and rights for the good of all. So all issues related to consent are critical for health professionals.

History of Consent

In early 1900; Sir Willium Osler, the father of modern medicine endorsed the necessity of informed consent in medical research. Till early 1930s; it was made clear by the Health Department regulations of Germany that both human experimentation and the use of novel treatment required consent in a clear and undebatable manner. Tuskegee Syphilis study is a famous example where innocent blacks were subjected to the inhuman studies following which President Clinton apologized in 1997.

Before the 20th century, guidelines required physician's need to adhere to acceptable medical standards. Issue of patient's agreement to the research never discussed. Most requirements arose after the Nuremberg trials.

Creation of Bioethics

Experiments during World War II and unethical clinical trials done by US Health Services gave birth of bioethics. It led to the creation of institutional review boards and notion of informed consent.

Informed Consent

Informed consent is a key instrument in protecting the right of the individual. Procurement of consent ensures human dignity of the participants and also shows respect for them. Informed consent is one of the primary ethical principles governing human subject research. Informed consent assures that prospective research subjects will understand the nature of the research and can knowledgeably and voluntarily decide whether or not to participate.

The fundamental ethical duty of respect for persons requires that we do not act against a person's wishes, and thus genuine consent to participate in research must be obtained.

WHAT CONSTITUTES INFORMED CONSENT?

Informed consent (Table 25.1) is a process and it involves providing all relevant information to the volunteer/patients. The patient/ volunteer understanding the information provided. The participants voluntarily agree to participate. This is considered to be a basic right. Guidelines for informed consent are given in Table 25.1.

CIOMS International Ethical Guidelines define informed consent as "consent given by a competent individual who has received the necessary information, has adequately understood the information, and after considering the information, has arrived at a decision without having been subjected to coercion, undue influence or inducement, or intimidation". Table 25.1 gives gross guidelines for informed consent.

Table 25.1: Guidelines for informed consent
- The Nuremberg code, 1947
- The Declaration of Helsinki, 1964 (2000)
- The Belmont Report, 1979
- ICH GCP, 1997
- ICMR Guidelines, 2000

WHY TO GET THE INFORMED CONSENT?

One would have to respect the person's autonomy and apply the principle of justice should something goes wrong in research. Informed consent is the first and longest of the 10 principles in the Nuremberg code. Informed consent is included in every guidelines on research ethics. It is also one of the 8 requirements for clinical research.

Informed consent allows individuals:
- To determine whether participating in research fits with their values and interests.
- To decide whether to contribute to this specific research project.
- To protect themselves from risks.
- To decide whether they can fulfill the requirements necessary for the research.

Providing Information in Informed Consent

Information provided in writing in the informed consent form should be discussed with the subject. Consent must be in a language the subject understands.

Nuremberg Code

This is a set of 10 principles on research involving humans. It was developed after the horrors of Nazi experiments on humans became public and was published in 1947. It mentions that the voluntary consent of the human subject is absolutely essential. Person must have legal capacity to consent. Also, the person should have "sufficient knowledge and comprehension" to make an "understanding and enlightened decision". Most importantly, person must be able to exercise "free power of choice".

One should inform the subject of the nature, duration and purpose of the research. Also the method and means of doing research should be mentioned. Person should have full knowledge of all inconveniences and hazards and their possible effects on health. There should be no force, fraud, deceit, duress, coercion.

The Declaration of Helsinki

This is a statement of ethical principles on research involving humans published by the World Medical Association. This has taken inspiration from Nuremberg code and some say it has borrowed heavily from the Nuremberg code. The best part is that it has been made by physicians. Also, it was first adopted at Helsinki in 1964.

It mentions that the subjects must be volunteers and/or informed participants. The consent should be obtained, preferably in writing. If the subject has a dependent relationship with the physician, consent should be obtained by an independent physician.

Consent is taken from legally acceptable representative required if the subject is a minor or is incapable of giving consent. Also if the physical or mental disability is present consent can be taken as a proxy consent.

When consent not possible prior to participation in research; then the work has to be approved by the "review committee". Consent must be obtained as soon as possible from the subject or a legally acceptable representative.

BELMONT REPORT

Belmont report is a set of ethical principles and guidelines for protecting humans in clinical research. It was developed by a commission set-up in the US in the aftermath of the Tuskeegee study becoming public and was published in 1979. Identifies three elements of the process, e.g. information about the research to the participants, comprehension so that they can understand and also the voluntariness.

Indian Council of Medical Research Guidelines (ICMR)

ICMR ethical guidelines for research involving humans were published under the theme, "Ethical Guidelines for Biomedical Research on Human Subjects" in year 2000.

The guidelines state that the participation in research must be voluntary and the participants must be "fully apprised of the research". The investigator must obtain informed consent and the responsibilities and information that must be provided to the subjects and investigators. Assent can be obtained, where possible, for minors. Requirement for consent can be waived by an ethics committee if risk is minimal, (e.g. collecting data from subjects' records), etc.

Bibliography

1. Consent process in trials. http://www.clinicaltrials.com/study_participants/informed_consent.htm (Downloaded February 9th 2017).
2. Consent taking in clinical trials. http://www.fda.gov/ForPatients/ClinicalTrials/InformedConsent/default.htm (Downloaded February 9th 2017).
3. Understanding informed consent in clinical trials. http://www.centerwatch.com/clinical-trials/understanding-informed-consent.aspx (Downloaded February 9th 2017).

Medical Ethics

Learning objective

There are various principles of research, such as beneficence, non-maleficence, autonomy, truth telling, confidentiality, preservation of life and justice. They need to be practiced in light of ethical principles. In modern world, it is crucial to have research that has sound ethical basis.

ETHICS IN RESEARCH

Ethics comes from Greek word *ethos* meaning thereby the morals of character. Ethics is a set of principles while the ethical committee is an independent body whose responsibility to ensure the protection of the rights, safety and well-being of human subjects involved in a trial and to provide public assurance of that protection. Composition of ethics committee is given in Table 26.1.

Three major functions of ethics
• Approval
• Ensure the protection of human subjects
• Periodic review

It ensure the study conducted as per the good clinical practice.

The research ethics committee is headed by a chairperson who is a man or woman of an

Table 26.1: Members in ethics committee

• Pharmacologist (basic medical scientist)
• Clinician
• Layperson
• Retired judge/advocate
• Social worker

impeccable integrity. The person will oversee the smooth functioning of ethics committee. There has to be at least four members present to be called a "meeting". The quorum is filled if at least five members are present.

How Ethics evolved?

The need for the ethical principles has long been felt. It had however been realized following the German "sea water experiments" and "high altitude experiments" that it is imperative to have some ethical regulations. The need was highlighted by the Tuskegee trial sponsored by the US Government where the blacks were exploited for alleged benefits that the scientific community were seeking. After this, the Belmont report of 1997, where it was clearly stated that there is need of a thorough review as to how the ethical principles could be evolved to benefit the mankind.

Institutional Review Board (IRB)

An independent body constituted of medical, scientific, and non-scientific members, whose responsibility is to ensure the protection of the rights, safety and well-being of human subjects involved in a trial by, among other things, reviewing, approving, and providing continuing review of trial protocol and amendments and of the methods and material to be used in obtaining and documenting informed consent of the trial subjects.

Ethics of Doing Medical Research in India

Ethics is made-up of the word *Ethos*, which is a Latin word meaning character. So character, like in all walks of life is very important in research. This is because, whenever a biomedical research project is undertaken; then there are issues that are relevant to safety of humans.

Over half a century ago, the concept of ethics in biomedical research was introduced. India is home to over a billion people and offers unique opportunity in clinical and biomedical research professionals. However, promoting ethics in biomedical research is vital to ensuring ethical use of vast number of patients' resource available with us. Without appropriate ethical considerations, whole of clinical and biomedical research involving patients will be in vein and even counter-productive. There is a need to introduce to ethical considerations, guidelines and recommendations for successful and worthwhile conduct of research among biomedical professionals.

History of Medical Ethics

It all started with war crimes where prisoners of wars were submersed in the cold water or made to fly at high altitude and it was noted that what was the end outcome. Therefore, the issues started erupting. The end point of many of these trials were death.

Likewise, there was an infamous syphilis experiment done in blacks and the explanations that they were given was that, "they had bad blood". On April 18th, 1879, Belmont report was published in the USA and subsequent to this; President of the US publically apologized for the ill behaviour of state doctors in handling the syphilis trial.

This prompted Nuremberg code that came into existence in 1949. This had several major principles that are still the backbone of clinical research:

1. Research participation should be voluntary.

2. Should be done by qualified persons.

3. Prior animal data must be there before human experiments could be done.

4. Good design should be there.

5. Patients or participants should have the freedom to opt out of the study whenever they feel like.

6. Minimal injury or risk should be there.

7. Investigator has to take the responsibility of the trial so that he or she could act as an inter-phase between ethics committee and the sponsors of the trial.

Some of the deficiencies of Nuremberg's code were brought out in the due course of time and were addressed by Helsinki's declaration. These guidelines were then adopted by World Medical Association 18th meeting and have been revised 6 times since then. Belmont report, discussed above had recommended three main principles of medical research:

1. Autonomy.

2. Beneficence.

3. Justice.

These three principles of research are valid even now and rather have become cornerstones.

WHY NEED SO MUCH OF REGULATION IN BIOMEDICAL RESEARCH?

The answer is simple! One would have to deal with humans. Not everyone is equipped with the medical knowledge and is familiar with terminology used. Therefore, some intervening agency had to be there, so that they could "protect" rights of the participants as well.

Though most clinical trials are done in accordance with clinical research protocols and violations are uncommon; still to protect the vulnerable sections of society, a body composed up of several sections of society is needed. Likewise, sponsors should have had exposed populations from other nationalities also to the drug and not just people from low income countries. More so, if a drug were to be used in the country where it is developed, it must be cost effective as well. So in nutshell, there are several issues.

Indian State in Ethics

Ethics is India started in 1980s, when first guidelines for Indian biomedical professionals were released. It was a small booklet of just 20 odd pages and guidelines were in their preliminary phase. Later in year 2000, the guidelines were revised and latest revision was done in 2006.

Discipline of medical ethics involving biomedical research in India is a relatively new phenomenon. Several medical colleges in India are yet to have their own ethical committees. Bioethics is yet to become a part of undergraduate curriculum. There are issues also about the way consent is obtained in clinical research. Table 26.2 gives chronology of medical ethics in India.

Table 26.2: Chronology of medical ethics evolution in India

1956—First small document released by Medical Council of India

1980—Policy statement on ethical consideration

1986—DNA handling guidelines

(Contd...)

Table 26.2: Chronology of medical ethics evolution in India *(Contd...)*

2000—Revised ethical guidelines

2001—Indian GCP guidelines

2002—Ammendement to Drugs and Cosmetic Act, Schedule-Y

2006—Revised ICMR guidelines

2013—Amendment to Drugs and Cosmetic Act, Schedule-Y

2014–2015—New guidelines circulated for comments

Bibliography

1. Basic ethical principles. https://www.med.uottawa.ca/sim/data/Ethics_e.htm (Downloaded February 9th 2017).
2. Code of medical ethics. https://www.ama-assn.org/about-us/code-medical-ethics (Downloaded February 9th 2017).
3. Medical ethics. https://www.ama-assn.org/about/medical-ethics (Downloaded February 9th 2017).

Intention to Treat Analysis

Learning objectives

Intention to treat analysis or ITT analysis refers to a statistical concept whereby study participants are analyzed according to the groups they were originally assigned to randomly, regardless of whether they dropped out or if they failed to comply with the treatment protocol allocated to their respective groups in the beginning of trial. So this means once randomized, "always analyzed". Inclusion in the ITT analysis should occur regardless of deviations that may happen after randomisation, such as protocol violations (e.g. those who received the comparator treatment or other treatments, rather than the allocated treatment), losses to follow up, withdrawals from the study, non-compliance or patients' refusal of the allocated treatment. It is important to know ITT analysis preserves the prognostic balance generated by the original random treatment allocation and this type of analysis is in contrast to 'per protocol' analysis and 'as treated' analysis.

Introduction

In the placebo controlled trials compliant patients who take their placebo have a better outcome (up to 30% better) than the non-compliant patients. If there is a large dropout in both the active and placebo arms of the trial it is attractive to analyse only those who received the active treatment (discarding the non-compliant patients in the active arm) but include all the patients entered into the placebo arm to increase the precision of the results. If the "active" treatment is actually of no benefit, because the non-compliant patients (who have worse outcomes) are only included in the placebo arm then the "active" treatment may falsely appear to be of benefit. ITT analysis removes this bias. ITT is an analysis in which patients are included in the group to which they were randomized irrespective of compliance, administrative errors (e.g. error in eligibility), or other protocol deviations.

Why do ITT Analysis: The Need?

In "real life" uptake of an intervention will never be "per-protocol" and hence, it is important to know that the intervention will still work, despite human error! Per protocol or PP analyses are based on a subset of participants. Results may not generalize to the population from which the original sample was taken. Reasons for attrition/non-adherence may be different across arms. Excluding people from the analysis accordingly may introduce confounding effects. The effect obtained via PP analysis reflects some combination of treatment effect and subset selection bias. It is impossible to disentangle the two PP analyses can also result in loss of power by reducing the number of observations available.

Whether ITT results in loss of power is an empirical question. In fact, studies have found that ITT analyses can result in larger treatment effects being observed than PP analyses. Hence, *planning* to not collect the data is not a solution. Halting data collection at treatment discontinuation may result in missing long-term effects of the treatment that arise even after treatment stops.

It is important to know that using ITT analysis helps improve retention protocols. One would have to develop a plan for missing data. Imputation, carrying last observation forward and instrumental variables, and other statistical techniques could be useful.

An additional option is to conduct secondary analyses. If data collection is stopped because of protocol non-adherence, then only PP analyses are possible. If participants contribute follow-up data irrespective of any protocol violation, both ITT and PP analyses can be performed.

What is Randomization?

Randomization for experimental studies was established by RA Fisher in 1923. International Conference on Harmonization (ICH) guidelines use the term "full analysis" set to refer to the set of all patients randomized.

Randomization can be viewed as a comparison of treatment protocols. Randomized control trials are an effective method for analyzing the efficacy and safety of two or more treatment options. Here subjects are randomly allocated groups receiving different interventions. The assignment occurs before any treatment or intervention is started. The benefit of this approach is that the groups only differ in terms of their intervention, hence reducing bias. Ideally all the subjects assigned to their respective groups would adhere to the treatment protocol and thus desired results will be generated. In practicality however, some subjects are unable to follow instructions or they might dropout of the study. Here the

statistical concept called ITT analysis helps overcome the problem.

Analysis of Randomized Trials

The primary analysis of randomized trials should be done via intention-to-treat analysis. To ensure that this analysis can be carried out, data collection following treatment discontinuation through the end of the trial should be a protocol requirement. Table 27.1 and Box 27.1 list the advantages and disadvantages of the same.

What are the Prerequisites of ITT Analysis?

For an efficient utilization of the ITT analysis technique, complete outcome data for all the subjects being randomly selected should be available. Care must be taken to minimize dropouts and maintain a close follow-up for all the subjects enrolled. This kind of set-up is perfect for utilization of ITT analysis technique. However, in case the study ends up missing some data, it can be dealt with using various methods as discussed further.

Dealing with Missing Data

There are four methods available for dealing with dropouts and missing data:
a. Complete-case analysis
b. Available-case methods

Table 27.1: Advantages and disadvantages of Intention to treat analysis

Pros	Cons
• ITT is supported by the CONSORT statement	• Estimate of treatment effect is conservative because of dilution due to noncompliance and more prone to Type 2 errors ('false negatives')
• It is more reliable estimate of true treatment effectiveness by replicating what happens in the 'real world'	
• Simplifies the task of dealing with suspicious outcomes as it includes all	• Heterogeneity is introduced when noncompliants, dropouts and compliant subjects are mixed together
• Prevents bias when incomplete data is related to outcome	• Does not assess treatment efficacy accurately unless there is negligible protocol violations, etc.
• Preserves baseline balance between groups	• Protocol violations and poorly conducted trials may cause the results obtained from two different treatment groups
• Minimises Type 1 errors ('false positives')	
• Preserves sample size (dropouts, etc. would otherwise decrease the sample size and decrease statistical power)	• ITT analysis alone is inappropriate for non-inferiority trials
• When the ITT and per-protocol analyses come to the same conclusions, confidence in the study results is increased	

Benefits:
- Preserves the sample size and maintains randomization
- Allows for generalizability and minimizes type I error
- Reflects a practical scenario

Drawbacks:
- Not a good method to determine the efficacy of treatment
- More caution required to maintain follow-up
- More susceptible to type II error

Methods to deal with missing data:
- Complete-case analysis
- Available-case methods
- Model-based approaches
- Imputation methods

Prerequisites:
- Complete outcome data should be available.
- Minimize dropouts and maintain a close follow-up

Alternative Techniques:
- Per-protocol (PP) analysis
- Treatment-received (TR) analysis

c. Model-based approaches
d. Imputation methods

Complete-case Analysis

The complete-case technique involves analyzing only those cases which went to completion and excluding the ones that dropped out or did not adhere to the treatment protocol. This method technically violates the concept of ITT analysis since a lot of data can go missing by excluding subjects thereby affecting the power of the study. In situations where dropouts are missing completely at random, this technique becomes valid.

Available-case Methods

The available-case technique comprises of a collection of methods which include repeated measurements of unequal length in the analysis. This technique utilizes the available data to compute statistical means and co-variances.

Model-based Approaches

The model-based approach is not a very widely used technique; it utilizes formal statistical methods to handle dropouts. They are based on certain assumptions which are not easily verifiable. Also, they are more time consuming and difficult to perform.

Imputation Methods

Imputation methods fill missing values in the data set. They are of two main types:
a. Fixed-value imputations
b. Multiple imputations

Fixed value imputations involve substituting all missing values with a fixed value. This fixed value is generated using various *ad hoc* techniques one of which is last observation carry forward method. This is the most widely used technique. It involves utilizing the last available value in the data set of a particular individual to fill in all the missing values for the same subject. Other *ad hoc* measures include the best value and worst value replacement techniques. In these techniques missing values are filled with the best value and the worst value respectively for the subject.

ITT Per Protocol/As-treated

This is an analysis in which patients are included in the group corresponding to the *treatment they actually received.* Patient compliance and "switchovers" are considered in the analysis. Typically, in PP analysis, patients who do not meet all of the eligibility criteria or do not adhere to the protocol are excluded, and events that occur after treatment discontinuation are excluded. ICH guidelines use the term PP to define a group of patients who were adherent to the protocol.

Steps for the Formal Design of a Study Using ITT

1. First of all a decision needs to be made if the study is pragmatic or explanatory. For pragmatic trials ITT analysis is very effective and necessary.
2. Decide on the inclusion criterion, violation of which would result in exclusion from the trial.

3. Try to minimize dropouts and maintain a close follow-up of subjects who withdraw from the treatment.

4. Incorporate all subjects allocated randomly to various groups. Also, compute the analysis after leaving out subjects who dropped out or did not follow the treatment protocol.

5. While reporting the final results make sure to mention that ITT analysis technique was utilized and also report all the missing responses. Discuss the potential effect of the missing data and derive conclusions based on ITT analysis.

Critical Analysis of Intention to Treat Analysis

The benefits of using ITT analysis are manifold. Firstly, it preserves the sample size and hence, the power of the study since it does not exclude noncompliant subjects or dropouts. Secondly, it reflects a practical scenario since it takes into account the possibility of people dropping out and not adhering to the advocated treatment. Thirdly, ITT analysis technique focuses on study design and conduct as well rather than just focusing on the analysis and the result part. Finally, it maintains randomization, allows for generalizability and also minimizes type I error.

The drawback of using ITT analysis technique is that it is not a good method to determine the efficacy of treatment since subjects who dropped out or did not adhere to the treatment protocol are also included in the final analysis. Also, interpretation of data might be difficult using this method in case a large proportion of subjects dropout or crossover to the other treatment arm. ITT analysis is more susceptible to type II error.

Modified ITT Concept

This technique differs from the classical one in the sense that subjects who are deemed ineligible after randomization or those who never started treatment in the first place are excluded from the analysis. Due to lack of consistent guidelines and involvement of a lot of subjectivity for entry criterion this technique

is deemed arbitrary and inaccurate involving a lot of bias. Modified ITT is mostly used for anti-infective trials where multiple populations are involved in a single study.

Alternatives to Using ITT Analysis

There are several alternatives to using ITT analysis. All of them have their strengths and weaknesses. Some of the techniques are discussed as below:

a. Per-protocol analysis

b. Treatment-received analysis

In the PP analysis, data from only those subjects who followed the protocol guidelines is analyzed. This is also referred to as "on treatment" analysis. One major drawback if this technique is that bias maybe introduced by excluding subjects from the study. Because of its limitations, ITT analysis should always be considered as the primary analysis technique supplemented by PP analysis.

Conclusion

In order to provide an unbiased analysis of a randomized control trial, the intention to treat analysis is an ideal technique to be utilized. In order to improve its applicability, investigators should attempt to minimize violation of study protocols and dropouts. In case of unavoidable circumstances where a close follow-up cannot be maintained various techniques to substitute missing data can be applied, however the results obtained using this method will not be as accurate.

Bibliography

1. Armitage P. Exclusions, losses to follow-up and withdrawals in clinical trials. In:Shapiro SH, Louis TA, editors. Clinical trials. New York: Marcel Dekker, 1983.

2. Bubbar VK, Kreder HJ. The intention-to-treat principle: A primer for the orthopaedic surgeon. J Bone Joint Surg Am. 2006; 88:2097–2099.

3. Deng CQ. Intention-to-Treat and modified Intention-to-Treat Analyses in Clinical Trials. PPD Development Research Triangle Park, NC 27560. [Last accessed on 2011 Jan 17].

4. Feinman RD. Intention-to-treat. What is the question? Nutr Metab (Lond) 2009; 6:1.

5. Fergusson D, Aaron SD, Guyatt G, Hébert P. Post-randomisation exclusions: The intention to treat principle and excluding patients from analysis. BMJ. 2002; 325:652–654.

6. Frangakis CE, Rubin DB. Addressing complications of intention-to-treat analysis in the combined presence of all-or-none treatment-noncompliance and subsequent missing outcomes. Biometrika. 1999; 86:365–379.

7. Gail MH. Eligibility, exclusions, losses to follow-up, removal of randomized patients and uncounted events in cancer clinical trials. Cancer Treat Rep.1985; 69: 1107–1113.

8. Heritier SR, Gebski VJ, Keech AC. Inclusion of patients in clinical trial analysis: The intention-to-treat principle. Med J Aust. 2003; 179:438–440.

9. Hollis S, Campbell F. What is meant by intention to treat analysis. Survey of published randomised controlled trials? BMJ. 1999; 319:670–674.

10. Iosief A, Alessandro M, Carlo R. Modified intention to treat: Frequency, definition and implication for clinical trials. 15th Cochrane Colloquium, Sao Paulo. 2007; 23–27.

11. Lewis JA, Machin D. Intention to treat—who should use ITT? Br J Cancer. 1993; 68:647–650.

12. Moher D, Schulz KF, Altman DG. CONSORT GROUP (Consolidated Standards of Reporting Trials). The CONSORT statement: Revised recommendations for improving the quality of reports of parallel-group randomized trials. Ann Intern Med. 2001; 134:657–662. [PubMed]

13. Moncur RA, Larmer JC. Clinical applicability of intention-to-treat analyses. MUMJ. 2009; 6:39–41.

14. Montori VM, Guyatt GH. Intention-to-treat principle. CMAJ. 2001; 165:1339–1341.

15. Peto R, Pike MC, Armitage P, et al. Design and analysis of randomized clinical trials requiring prolonged observation of each patient. Br J Cancer 1976; 34: 585–612.

16. Sainani KL. Making sense of intention-to-treat. PM R. 2010; 2:209–213.

17. Sally Hollis S, Fiona Campbell F. What is meant by intention to treat analysis? Survey of published randomised controlled trials. BMJ. 1999 Sep 11; 319(7211): 670–674.

18. Soares I, Carneiro AV. Intention-to-treat analysis in clinical trials: Principles and practical importance. Rev Port Cardiol. 2002; 21:1191–1198.

19. Ten Have TR, Normand SL, Marcus SM, Brown CH, Lavori P, Duan N. Intent-to-Treat vs. Non-Intent-to-Treat Analyses under Treatment Non-Adherence in Mental Health Randomized Trials. Psychiatr Ann. 2008; 38:772–783.

20. Touloumi G, Babiker AG, Pocock SJ, Darbyshire JH. Impact of missing data due to drop-outs on estimators for rates of change in longitudinal studies: a simulation study. Stat Med. 2001; 20:3715–3728.

21. Unnebrink K, Windeler J. Intention-to-treat: methods for dealing with missing values in clinical trials of progressively deteriorating diseases. Stat Med. 2001; 20:3931–3946.

22. Wertz RT. Intention to treat: Once randomized, always analyzed. Clin Aphasiol. 1995; 23: 57–64.

28 Number Needed to Treat (NNT), Number Needed to Harm (NNH), Hazard Ratios

Learning objectives

Number needed to treat (NNT) is an interesting concept. It means, if a drug under clinical development has NNT as 10 then it would mean that we shall have to treat 10 people to be able to prevent 1 bad outcome. Likewise, number needed to harm is similar to NNT and indicates how many patients need to be exposed to a risk factor to cause harm in one patient (e.g. how many men must be smoking for 1 patient to have lung cancer), who in the absence of smoking will not develop lung cancer.

NUMBER NEEDED TO TREAT (NNT)

Number Needed to Treat or NNT is a statistical concept but is intuitive too. We know that when a new drug comes and is used for patients; not everyone is helped or benefited. Some are helped, some are harmed, some unaffected too. NNT tells us how many of each!

This is the average number of persons who would have to receive an intervention for 1 to benefit. Ideally, NNT should be 1 as everyone should benefit in an ideal world!

The opposite is known as Number Needed to Harm (NNH), which is the number of persons who would have to receive an intervention for 1 to be experience an adverse event.

WHY ESTIMATE NNT?

This is simile method to know if a treatment of a drug will help a given person. It can easily be calculated from the results of a trial.

HOW TO CALCULATE NNT?

To be fair, both harms and benefits should be presented in absolute terms or relative terms.

Number needed to treat is an important means of evaluating data. NNT is calculated by taking the reciprocal of the absolute difference (absolute risk reduction) between experimental groups (experimental and control groups). Another way is by dividing 100 by absolute risk.

Follow this example: If a disease has a mortality of 100% without treatment and therapy reduces that mortality to 50%, how many people would you need to treat to prevent 1 death? The answer is 2 patients.

Usefulness of NNT

Number needed to treat is one way to communicate the effectiveness of a treatment. It is growing in popularity and is often reported in randomized control trials and systematic reviews on therapy. It signifies how many patients would need to be treated to get one additional patient better who would not have gotten better without this particular treatment.

An NNT of 10 for treating otitis media with antibiotics indicates that 10 patients need to be given an antibiotic to get one more patient better than would have improved without the antibiotics. It does not reflect how many patients get better in total. The other nine are probably a combination of patients who would have gotten better even without treatment and perhaps some that did not get better despite the antibiotic (e.g. they may have had an allergic sinusitis). This method offers one convenient way to think about how good a particular treatment is.

WHAT IF NNT IS NOT GIVEN?

If a paper does not report the NNT, but does report the absolute risk (AR), the NNT can be easily calculated. For example, if 80% of patients in the control group got better and 90% of patients in a treatment group got better, the absolute risk of not getting better if denied the more effective treatment is 10%.

In other words, the absolute risk reduction (ARR) is 10% (0.1). The NNT will be 1/0.1 = 10. That means, for every 10 patients who get this treatment, 1 more would get better compared to the control group.

Pitfalls of NNT

An NNT tells about how many patients would benefit, but it does not tell you how much they may benefit or a number of other key factors. Beware of reading or citing NNTs without knowing the context.

Here are some things that one would need to know about the NNT to help judge its worth better: What defined treatment success? Complete cure?

A 30% improvement (that probably is clinically significant)? A 5% improvement in pain (probably not considered clinically significant)?

What was it compared to? Placebo? Another therapy that's known to be effective? Or no treatment?

- How long did the results last (what was the length of follow-up)?
- What phase was the injury in (acute, subacute? chronic?)
- How severe was the condition?

WHAT IS A GOOD NNT?

A perfect NNT would be 1. That means that for very patient treated one got better in the study who would not have otherwise without that particular intervention.

It is hence clear that the larger the number, the fewer people will be helped. What one considers a "good enough" NNT is going to be a judgment call based not only on the NNT itself but also on a carefully balanced consideration the following like how robust

the treatment outcome is (does it completely cure the patient or just make them a small percentage better?) or the cost (is it expensive?)

The risk of treatment like if the side effects are common or not? What is the probability of serious adverse events and if there is a better treatment available or not?

Putting NNTs into Perspective

As a general rule of thumb, an NNT of 5 or under for treating a symptomatic condition is usually considered to be acceptable and in some cases even NNTs below 10.

Hazard Ratios

This is a common expression in clinical trials. A hazard ratio considers the absolute risk as 1. If something lowers the risk, e.g. anti-diabetics reducing the risk of stroke by 30%; the hazard ratio is 0.7, i.e. one would still face the risk to the tune of 70%. Eating lot of sweets, not exercising and remaining sedentary may increase the risk of stroke by 3 times so the hazard ratio will be 3.0.

Hazard ratio is ratio of hazards in two groups and remains constant overtime. The Cox Proportional Hazards model is the most used analytical tool in survival research.

Cox Proportional Hazard Model

One should understand the general form of Cox Proportional Hazard Model. Also the need for adjusted Hazard Ratios (HR) (Figs 28.1 to 28.3).

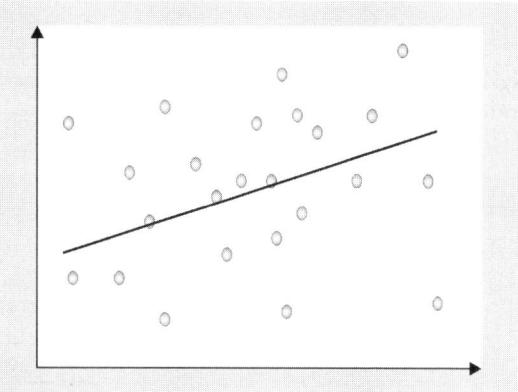

Fig. 28.1: One of the major aim of cox modeling is to be able to identify "signal from noise"

Hazard ratio is expressed in terms of the hazard function formally defined as: the instantaneous risk of event (mortality) in next time interval t, conditional on having survived to start of the interval t.

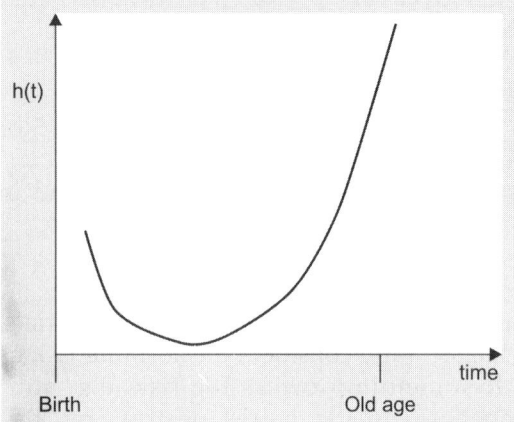

Fig. 28.2: Hazard rate is an instantaneous rate of events as a function of time. Note that the hazard changes overtime denoted by h(t)

The Cox model expresses the relationship between the hazard and a set of variables or covariates, e.g. age, gender, social deprivation, Dukes stage of cancer, comorbidity, etc.

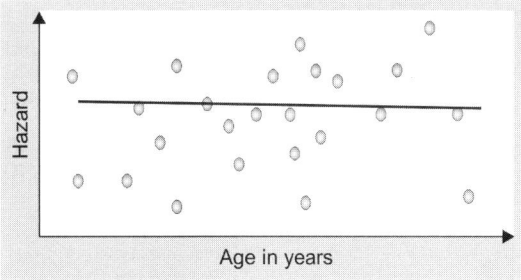

Fig. 28.3: Graphical representation of hazard function and age in years

The simples equation is develops when (h) is the hazard (K) is a constant ($h = k$).

A linear equation can be constructed: h is the outcome; a is the intercept; β is the slope related to x the explanatory variable and; e is the error term or 'noise'.

$$h = a + \beta x + e_i$$

h_0 is the baseline hazard; r (β, x) function reflects how the hazard function changes (β) according to differences in subjects' characteristics (x).

$$h\,(t) + H_0\,(t) \times r\,(\beta, x)$$

Interpreting Hazard Ratio

HR = 1; Do not reject null hypothesis (i.e. no difference).

HR < 1; Reduction in hazard relative to comparator (e.g. HR = 0.6 is 40% reduction).

HR > 1; Increase in hazard relative to comparator (e.g. HR = 1.7 is 70% increase).

Bibliography

1. Andrade C. The numbers needed to treat and harm (NNT, NNH) statistics: what they tell us and what they do not. J Clin Psychiatry. 2015 Mar;76(3):e330–3. doi: 10.4088/JCP. 15f09870.

2. NNT explained. http://www.thennt.com/ thennt-explained/(Downloaded on May 4th 2017).

3. The numbers needed to treat and harm http:// www.bmj.com/content/341/bmj.c5731 (Downloaded on May4th 2017).

Evidence-Based Medicine

Learning objectives

Evidence medicine is explicit, judicious use of modern medicine to make clinical judgment about the individual patients. This integrates clinical experience and patient values with best available research information.

Evidence-Based Medicine (EBM) means current best evidence integrates with clinical expertise, pathophysiological knowledge and patient preference to make healthcare decisions. In recent times, emphasis on evidence-based medicine has increased. Particularly, in last 10 years or so, this has been on the move. Ever since its definition around 50 years back, it has been adopted by major organizations like Cochrane collaborations and centre for evidence-based medicine (Fig. 29.1).

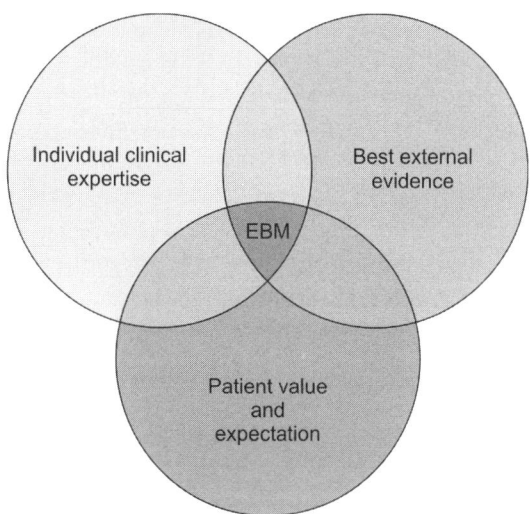

Fig. 29.1: Triad of EBM. Note that it combines clinical experience of doctors and evidence-based evidence from trials and also patients' expectations, so all stakeholders in EBM fit in comfortably

Table 29.1: Levels of evidence (United States Preventive Services Task Force for ranking evidence, 1989)

- **Level I evidence:** Evidence obtained from at least one properly designed randomized controlled trial.

- **Level II-1 evidence:** Evidence-obtained from well-designed controlled trials without randomization.

- **Level II-2 evidence:** Evidence-obtained from well-designed cohort or case-control analytic studies, preferably from more than one center or research group.

- **Level II-3 evidence:** Evidence-obtained from multiple time series designs with or without the intervention. Surprising results in uncontrolled trials might also be regarded as this type of evidence.

- **Level III evidence:** Opinions of respected authorities, based on clinical experience, or reports of expert committees.

The process starts with defining question → search literature → integrate the same in practice.

WHY NEED EBM?

This has been developed to bridge the gap between research and practice. In gone by era, experience was the key, likewise now there is an era of EBM. This is aimed at integrating both the science and art in medicine-based on available evidence (Tables 29.1, 29.2, and Fig. 29.2).

Table 29.2: Advantages of EBM

Interpretation of literature is easy

Provides objective basis of therapy selection

Modifies practice

Gaps in knowledge filled

Disease management becomes easily

Table 29.3: Levels of recommendations (United States Preventive Services Task Force for ranking evidence, 1989)

- **Level A:** Good evidence suggesting benefits of the clinical service substantially outweigh the potential risks.
- **Level B:** Fair evidence suggests that the benefits of the clinical service outweighs the potential risks.
- **Level C:** Fair evidence suggests that there are benefits provided by the clinical service, but the balance between benefits and risks are too close for making general recommendations. Clinicians need not offer it unless there are individual considerations.
- **Level D:** Fair evidence suggests that the risks of the clinical service outweighs potential benefits. Clinicians should not routinely offer the service to asymptomatic patients.
- **Level I:** Scientific evidence is lacking, of poor quality, or conflicting, such that the risk versus benefit balance cannot be assessed.

Though experience of clinicians is important but decisions based on experience alone may not be reliable. Therefore, there has to be an objective basis of selecting therapies. Likewise, physicians who have a good knowledge of pathophysiology will do better than the ones who do not have, but this too may not be sufficient. Integrating clinical experience with such knowledge coupled with experience may be a better approach.

In recent times, however, emphasis is on finding evidence that one type of treatment is superior to the other. This is done with help of clinical trials. Notably, clinical trials are the highest form of evidence and provide best

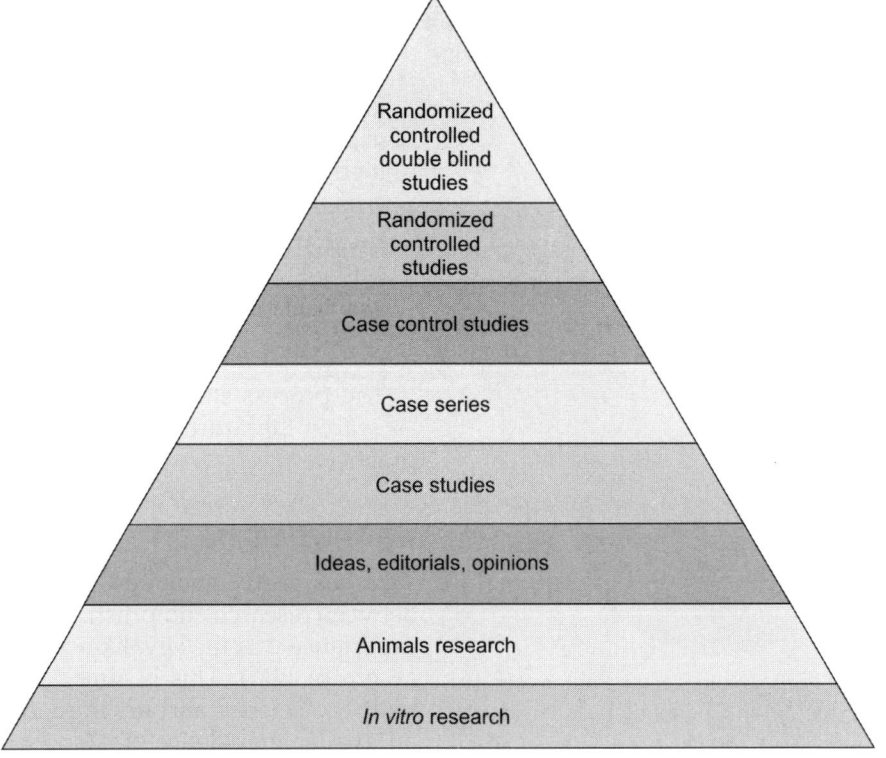

Fig. 29.2: Hierarchy of clinical research. Note that higher up we go, better evidence emerges

evidence of clinical judgment. EBM has helped to remove subjective bias.

EBM has also helped to integrate various types of data, e.g. clinical, pathophysiological and helps in objective analysis as well. The best part is that integration of all available information to take sound and better clinical decisions (Table 29.4).

Table 29.4: A quick guide to select the best research design and its property

Level of evidence	Study design	Status
I	RCT	Gold standard, equal probability of assignment
II	Cohort studies	Exposure is important in definition
III	Case control studies	Defined by outcome of interest
IV	Case series	Uncontrolled studies
V	Expert opinion	Depends upon quality of expert

Statistical Methods used in EBM

Likelihood Ratio

Both pre-test and post-test odd can be converted into probability which is easier to interpret.

Receiver-operator Curve (ROC)

In this type of curve, the true positive rate or sensitivity (the diseased individuals) is plotted as the function of false positive rate (healthy or 100-specifity) for different cut-off. Each point on ROC represents a sensitivity/specificity pair to a particular decision point threshold (Fig. 29.3).

Number Needed to Treat

This is a way of expressing effectiveness and safety of a clinical intervention. It is always computed with regards to two treatment. A defined endpoint has to be specified. For example, if an investigation, hypothetically speaking if a test has a NNT of 300, then one has to screen 300 cases before finding a positive case. If a treatment has a NNT of four,

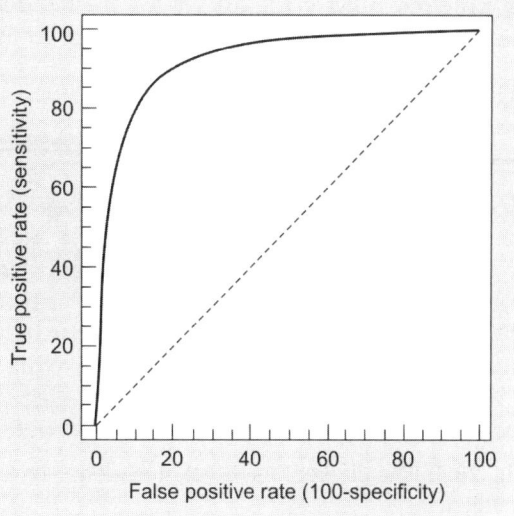

Fig. 29.3: Receiver operator characteristic curve (ROC)

that means, four cases need to be treated to get one clinically useful outcome (Fig. 29.4).

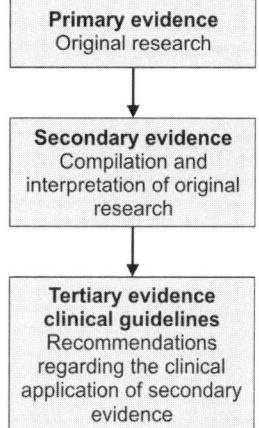

Fig. 29.4: Evaluation of research paper involves critical analysis

Evaluating a Research Paper

Criticism of EBM

EBM produces results in a quantitative manner. Therefore, the results cannot be applied to all treatments or situations. Sometimes, treatment efficacy reported in clinical trials may be different from effectiveness or real life usefulness of clinical trial. However, in present situations, despite limitations, there is no substitute of EBM. Note that to be able to practice EBM critically, 5-As are needed (ask, acquire, act, appraise, apply) (Fig. 29.5).

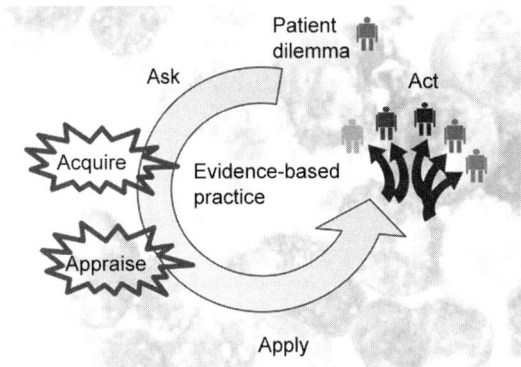

Fig. 29.5: Five different As (5-As) of evidence-based medicine

Bibliography

1. Evidence Based Medicine. http://med. fsu. edu/index.cfm?page=medicalinformatics. ebmTutorial (Downloaded on May 4th 2017).

2. Izet Masic, Milan Miokovic, and Belma Muhamedagic. Evidence Based Medicine– New Approaches and Challenges. Acta Inform Med. 2008; 16(4): 219–225.

3. United States Preventive Services Task Force for ranking evidence about the effectiveness of treatments or screening. US Preventive Services Task Force (August 1989). Guide to clinical preventive services: report of the US Preventive Services Task Force. DIANE Publishing. pp. 24–. ISBN 978-1-56806-297-6.

Recent Advances in Medical Research Administration in India

Learning objectives

Growth of clinical/medical research in India has been significant in last few years. In medical research, clinical trials are being conducted at a rapid pace. Hence one needs to familiarize oneself about the changing scenario.

Introduction

Clinical research has grown exponentially over the past decade in India because of several reasons (Table 30.1).

Table 30.1: India advantages in clinical research

- Cost advantage
- Qualified doctors conversant in English
- Trained manpower

Clinical Research in India as it Stands

India was the second most preferred country to conduct clinical trials outside the US in 2009. However, recent years have witnessed a decline in number of trials in India (529 in 2010; 253 in 2012). The number of drugs entering the Indian markets had been gradually reducing even before the current slump in clinical research activity (270 in 2008; 140 in 2011; 44 in 2012 and 25 in 2013). It has been suggested that this necessitates a relook on the strategy so as to optimize clinical research in Indian context and take best advantage of available opportunities in this area.

Challenges: Need for Training

The problems and possibilities around the clinical research can be broadly grouped as:

a. **Growth:** Capacity building issues are an urgent need as to increase the quality and quantity of clinical research professionals in India.

b. **Ethical/regulatory:** Ethical committee could be made more robust and proactive in screening clinical trials. However, they should not hamper the progress of science and be the guardians of human rights. In India, Drug Controller General India (DCGI) is the competent authority for approving clinical trials as well as manufacturing and marketing drugs. DCGI grants approval after appropriate clinical trials are conducted in India with adequate number of trial subjects. As the number of clinical trials waiting to be approved increase if India were to take the leadership role, then the capacity building and issues and swiftness may need to be addressed. Though India has a robust regulatory framework, it is often perceived that Indian patients being poor and less informed and are vulnerable. While isolated instances of unethical clinical trials cannot be ignored, a more informed debate and perception management is the need of the hour. Heavy regulation in clinical research is potentially preventive.

c. **Training:** There are scant training resources to train adequate number of researchers so as to carry out research activities as per the international standards. There is a need to build dynamic training modules and platforms which confirm to international regulations and best practices while addressing peculiar national needs. The training infrastructure needs to be flexible enough to accommodate ever changing regulatory recruitments.

d. **Traditional medicine research:** India has a good knowledge base of traditional medicine systems which cater to a large segment of the population are regulated by a separate department of traditional medicines (e.g. AYUSH). There is a requirement of involving AYUSH practitioners in collaborative research and reorient the research regulations so as to effectively monitor research in AYUSH. Recent draft regarding regulations for herbal medicines is a positive step in this direction.

e. **Confidence building:** The confidence building amongst all stakeholders has now assumed paramount importance. Lot of steps to ensure participant safety by introducing major changes in regulatory framework of clinical research in India have been taken recently. Some such changes are as follows.

f. **Registration of clinical trials:** Registration of clinical trials of all clinical trials with Clinical Trial Registry India (CTRI) is mandatory with effect from February, 2013. The protocol, enrollment and the final report also need to be uploaded at the registry. This is a welcome step aimed at putting trial related information in the public domain. However, there is a case for broadening the ambit of CTRI by capturing the subsequent trial results (positive, negative or inconclusive termination) too in the national database. This step shall go a long way in ensuring optimum publicity of trial results thereby mitigating publication bias.

g. **Audio-visual consent:** From June, 2013, an audio-visual recording of the informed consent process is now mandatory to make the process more transparent and maintaining confidentiality. Reservations on logistics of this notification has been expressed by stakeholders, however amendments are awaited. Till the time,

it becomes a commonplace, some questions remain.

h. **Institutional committee registration:** Registration of Institutional Ethics Committees (IECs) is mandatory with effect from February, 2013. IECs have been empowered and made more accountable. Now, they are required to actively monitor and participate in reporting of SAEs. Strict timelines for reporting of Serious Adverse Events (SAEs) have been mandated in which IEC has to give their report including opinion on compensation within a fixed time frame. Investigators are required to report SAEs to the IEC within 24 hours followed by a detailed report within 14 days. Within next 30 days, IECs have to analyse and forward these reports to national expert committee with opinion on financial compensation. In order to fulfill their responsibility, IEC should be competent. Therefore training of IECs needs to be undertaken so as to empower them about their roles and responsibilities.

i. **Financial compensation:** Financial compensation based on no—fault principle calculated as per defined formula has been made the mandatory responsibility of the sponsor for trial related injuries or death. This comprehensive and dynamic formula has been so devised that younger participants get more compensation as compared to older participants. The final order regarding compensation is given by the DCGI which has to be complied within 30 days. If the trial related injury is discerned after the completion of trial, still the compensation has to be given. The financial compensation to be paid is over and above free medical management of injury that has to be provided to the participant. In addition, trial participants have to be provided ancillary care if they suffer from for any other illness during the trial. The calculation of compensation for trial related injury is derived from the one applicable in case of trial related deaths. It is based on the assumption that death is the maximum injury possible to an individual and the amount in case of injury has to be less than the amount that would have been applicable in case of death in similar circumstances. According to this formula, the trial related SAEs for deciding the amount of compensation have been divided into following four categories—permanent disability; congenital anomaly or birth defect, chronic life-threatening disease; or reversible SAE in case it is resolved. The compensation applicable in all these scenarios has to be calculated differently.

k. **Accreditation of principal investigators:** Principal investigators, ethical committees and the trial sites accreditation has been recommended to ensure competence of investigator(s), IEC members and the capacity of the site.

Recent Developments

Besides the regulatory action, patient, the most important stakeholder, needs to be sensitized too. There is a need to generate informed and balanced debate in electronic and print media. The entire spectrum of clinical research needs to be made transparent with seamless knowledge sharing and information exchange. Regulators also need to act more as facilitators of research and not merely as law enforcers. The regulations have been made after detailed deliberations, consultations and analysis of the situation. These steps were essential to fill the gaps in the regulations, in absence of which there can be potential harm to the trial participants, who are relatively less informed as compared to their counterparts in the developed world. However, it is perceived that at few points, there is some over-correction which needs to be adjusted based on the evidence and detailed discussion with all the stakeholders, so that the progress of science is also not affected. While the arena of clinical trials is under close watch, other types of clinical research, such as observational studies, population based studies, outcomes research, etc. also deserve equal emphasis.

We need to formulate standardized protocols for these activities and train adequate manpower. In the country of our size and magnitude, this is where the clues and leads are likely to emerge from.

Another important issue is to align the clinical research activity in our country as per our national health needs. Research in India specific problems (such as encephalitis, dengue, malaria, tuberculosis) should be incentivized by way of faster approvals, liberal funding and extended marketing rights. It is good to have a vaccine against HPV but one against encephalitis may be needed more and sooner.

Need of Clinical Research in India

Clinical research is essential not only for developing medicines for emerging health concerns that India faces day in and day out (such as XDR TB, antibiotic resistant pathogens, H_1N_1, Ebola virus, etc.) but also for finding safer and better medicines for entrenched diseases, such as HIV, malaria, diabetes, hypertension, etc. India, with its large patient population, unmet health needs, and limited resources, needs to make newer and better treatment options available to its population in a quick, economical and dependable manner. For this, India must take proactive part in clinical research and assume leadership role globally. It must be ensured that clinical research in India is carried out as per global scientific standard, is moored in sound ethical foundations befitting a liberal democracy but is optimally oriented towards addressing national medical and health needs.

Bibliography

1. Clinical research in India. http://www. excellifesciences.com/clinical-research-india/ (Accessed online July 3rd, 2017).

2. Clinical trial industry in India. http://isid. org.in/pdf/WP179.pdf (Accessed online May 5th, 2017).

3. Growth of clinical research in India. http:// www.clinnex.com/clinical-research/4-reasons-why-clinical-research-in-india-is-all-poised-for-growth-in-2017/(Accessed online May 5th, 2017).

4. Healthcare research and industry in India. https://www.ibef.org/industry/healthcare-india.aspx (Accessed online May 5th, 2017).

5. http://www.financialexpress.com/article/pharma/management-pharma/current-status-of-clinical-research-in-india/51148/ (Accessed online July 3rd, 2015).

6. India is poised to gain from clinical research. http://timesofindia.indiatimes.com/business/india-business/Indias-attractive-again-for-clinical-trials-Quintiles-CEO/articleshow/51716878.cms (Accessed online July 3rd, 2017).

Present Effectively

Learning objectives

Presenting the topics effectively is an art and needs practice and experience. One would have to show passion and interest towards the audience and be able to connect as well. One would have to focus on the needs of participants. Additionally, the topic should be kept simple while the core message should be emphasized. Eye to eye contact with the audience is a must. Starting of the topic should be good to be able to gain momentum. Telling short stories makes topic interesting. Slides should not be far too many and should not be containing lot of material. Take home message should be given in the end.

Introduction

Scientific presentations are commonplace and all people in biomedical sciences have to present something or other at one point of time or other. There are no set rules for effective presentations and varies from individual to individuals. However, there are 3 Ps of effective presentations (**Prepare, Planning** and **Presentations**).

Prepare

One of my professors of neurology always used to say, "Prepare well before you go to a scientific presentation. This is an important aspect of the whole exercise (Fig. 31.1 and Table 31.1).

Importantly, people who are ill prepared may not be able to leave any impression on their audiences, on the other hand the people who ware well prepared will an indelible impressions. Therefore, preparations are the first and foremost aspect of an scientific presentation.

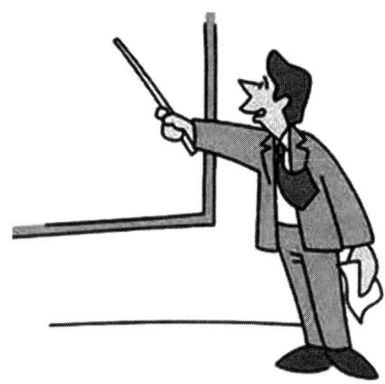

Fig. 31.1: Good preparations always help. It increases the confidence of the presenter and also arouses the interest and attention of the listeners. One of the major problems in presentations comes when the presenter assumes that the audiences know everything

Table 31.1: Prerequisite of preparing

- Know the topic well.
- Read latest information.
- Organize the talks.
- Do not be fast, rehearse well.
- Avoid long sentences in the slides.
- Avoid abbreviations. This may confuse listeners.
- Plan in such a manner, that at your speed, you will be able to finish in time.
- Do not use complicated tables. More than four columns could be a lot!
- Pie charts are always better than the columns as they are read easily.
- Avoid putting lot of text.
- Consult a doctor, if you have stage fear!

Planning

Failing to plan, is planning to fail: One should be able to organize the transcript in such a way, that it is effectively delivered. Planning stage would include a number of things, e.g. your audience, their levels, and also their interest in the topic. Remember, in a scientific meeting, there will always be people from varied background and hence, the planning should be done keeping the mutual interest in mind. For example, in a lecture on dementias; one could expect MSc, PhDs, MDs and DMs and hence, the planning should be done keeping the interest of all of these people in mind. Failure at this stage leads to disinterest and the effeteness of presentation may be compromised. A very common error is when someone overshoots the allotted time and goes on and the chairpersons have to press buzzers to stop the presentation! This is embarrassing so, keep in mind time allotted! Remember; in planning stage itself know your speed and the time in which you could deliver the same content. Good rehearsals are always handy and will allow one to be able to deliver the content effectively (Table 31.2).

Table 31.2: Prerequisite of planning

- Know your audience well
- Their level of knowledge
- Interest
- Motivation
- Level of understanding
- Keep in mind time allotted

Presentation

In the real presentation, one should keep in mind 3 worlds-3s, i.e. select, synthesize and simplify. One of the common error that may presenters do in beginning is that "they just read the power point presentations". In the beginning, start with something general, say about the place you been visiting and the hospitality you got. This may help to warm up the audience. Additionally, you may also add a "punch line" that will help your audience. Such a simple exercise may increase

the attention of audience to a great deal and they get more interested if they know the importance of the subject (Table 31.3).

Table 31.3: Prerequisite of presentations

- Write lines (4–6 lines) per slide.
- Do not give excuses "this is busy slide" very often.
- Know your audience well (refer preperations).
- Do not just read the slides.
- Do not turn away from the audience and focus on slides themselves.
- Face up to the audience, but do not look at a particular face.
- Give equal attention to the audiences.
- Try to avoid long explanations and get stuck to one slide or a point.
- Refrain from putting hands in the pocket or be rigid in your posture.
- Stay relaxed, dress comfortably.
- If formal dress, improves your confidence, so be it.
- Include pictures and text in the slides.
- Use cartoons for simplification.
- Use a minute on each slide if you have information to tell and 5–10 seconds/slides if this needs to told and not explained.
- Hold the interest of the audience and keep it lighthearted. Keeping it too didactic can put audiences off.

Visual aids are very important aspect of the presentations. It is often said that we just remember 20% of what we hear but this increases to 30%, if we see. Now, if we see and hear both; then it can increase to 50%. Therefore, a combination of "hear and see" is more effective than just seeing and hear alone. If you are lucky to have a good and receptive audience, this "see and hear" percentage may increase to 75%. In author's experience, if the individuals are made to "work" also along with hear and see, then the percentage of learning is much better. So Chinese saying, "picture is worth thousand words" is applicable here. In general, visual aids help the following:

a. Hold attention of the audience.
b. Avoid the need of using text.
c. Deliver the message in simple manner.

Warming up and Getting Started

This is very important and if the warm-up has been good; then the tone for the presentation is set. Long explanations about why you were here and how was the weather of the place attracting your attention and the food at local restaurants has interested you or the beauty of the town enthralled you, may put audience off! All this should be summarized in shortest possible words and one should get down to business quickly (Fig. 31.2).

a. "Feel" that you read the topic and know your topic well. Do not assume that your audience will know more about the topic.

b. Avoid being overconfident, this can put you in trouble when senior listeners are sitting.

c. Always start with a welcome note, like, "Good morning all" or "Good evening" rather than starting abrupt. It is handy, to give a brief introduction of the events.

d. Look at your transcript. If you have a 10 minute presentation; then your transcript should not have more than 5 pages double space text 12 font size, times new roman.

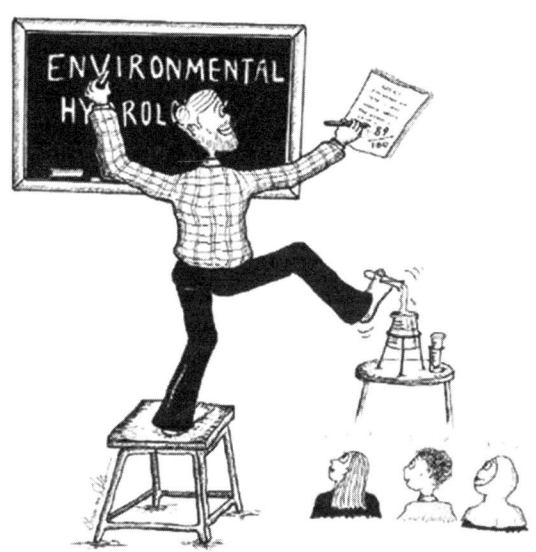

Fig. 31.2: Dressing formally and be calm and composed helps. The gestures that we use to explain will also get the attention of audiences. Remember you are being watched. A too causal presenter is unlikely to get the attention they rightfully deserve

e. You can thank the organizers or your professor if he or she is also present. Remember, you have been trained by someone. You do not loose anything by expressing your gratitude (Fig. 31.3).

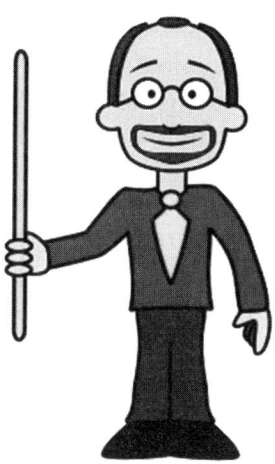

Fig. 31.3: Do not be rigid. Handle questions gently and appreciate audience if they do well. This is particularly good if you presenting something for undergraduates or junior grade classes

f. One should be gentle in handling questions if they are asked. Appreciating a good question is always helpful. One should appreciate the sharp responses given by audiences. Asking too many questions would turn your audiences from "attentive" to "anxious". Avoid asking questions after every other slide. Audience appreciates if there is an uncommon aspect you brought to their notice and if someone out of them knew the answer, it can be handy.

In general, presentations are done using the power point slides. These are of three different types:

1. Text slides
   a. Do not make them crowded.
   b. Use few and short sentences
   c. "Use key points"
   d. Do not tell a lot that is not written in slides.
   e. Also never read the ditto copy, your audience can read that as well.

Remember, you not a reader of Power Point slides; rather you are there to teach or share your experience.

2. Data slides.
    a. Figures
        i. Use simple figures.
        ii. Do not use tables that have several columns.
        iii. Readable lines should be used as a legend rather than very small.
    b. Diagrams
        i. Should be self-explanatory.
        ii. Scatter diagrams are good to show the relationships.
        iii. Flow diagrams should be simple.
3. Pictures
    a. Avoid too many pictures.
    b. Colors in presentations are used to enhance understanding.
    c. Unnecessary decoration could confuse the audience.
    d. One could include the animations and videos; make sure you have checked them well before going out. Remember, "pendrive" or "harddisck" malfunctions will put the audiences off. Prepare well.
    e. If you are presenting in some smaller city of India; where power back-up facility may not be very good; be prepared deal with this. That means, over-reliance on the Power Point presentations could be problematic in some situations.

Some of the presenters are very comfortable with the overhead presentations (OHPs).

They offer several advantages
    a. Good for small group.
    b. Presenter can face up to the audience rather than towards the board.
    c. Give a feel of "live class" where the presenter can write something on the OHP transparencies. Moreover, they provide a good method if a teacher were to take the class with junior students.

Disadvantages are
    a. Not suitable for large audiences.
    b. Sharpness of writing may be missing.

    c. If not neatly prepared, they may give an impression of "bad presentation".
    d. If you have bad handwriting, then the printed slides could be used. These are much better and give the audience a chance to understand better. Printers now can print directly on slides. During presentations, one could use the pen to write directly on the transparency.

Summary

Effective presentation is an art and comes with time. However, simple rules like getting ready, reaching before time, getting to know your computers and instruments and be comfortable with podium are general rules. Additionally, observe the following:

- Do not come late.
- Do not blame organizers if something goes wrong.
- Manage your slides.
- Keep up to time.
- Avoid spontaneity.
- Prepare well before you come.
- Rehearse well.
- Use your own style of speaking rather than a copied one.
- Stick to the topic you have been given for presentation rather than some else.
- If you have presented something and has invited questions also; perhaps is a good presentation. No questions at all may not be a good sign.
- Do not forget to say, "Does that answer your question?" if someone has asked.

Happy presentations!

Bibliography

1. Delivering an effective presentation. http://www 2.le.ac.uk/offices/ld/resources/presentations/delivering-presentation (Downloaded on May 4th 2017).
2. Tips for effective presentations. https://www.skillsyouneed.com/present/presentation-tips.html (Downloaded on May 4th 2017).
3. Present effectively. https://www.inc.com/geoffrey-james/how-to-fix-your-presentations-21-tips.html (Downloaded on May 4th 2017).

Meta-analysis in Medical Research

Learning objectives

Meta-analysis are the studies of the randomized trials that provide a precise estimate of the treatment effects. These give due weightage to the size of the "treatment difference" included. The validity of meta-analysis depends upon the quality of systematic review on which it is based. Good meta-analysis aims to have complete coverage of all relevant studies and look for the presence of heterogeneity. These also explore the robustness of the main findings using sensitivity analysis. Their popularity has grown a lot in recent times due to their superiority over the systematic and traditional reviews. Though considered to be "desk jobs" by the clinicians but are among the most exciting works done in clinical research whose results are directly relevant to clinical practice.

What is Meta-analysis?

Meta-analysis is a statistical technique for combining the findings from independent studies and is often used to assess the clinical effectiveness of healthcare intervention. This is done by combining the two or more randomized control studies. Meta-analysis offers a rational and helpful way of dealing with a number of practical difficulties that beset anyone trying to make sense of effectiveness research.

Basically, meta-analysis is a statistical process of combining data from several studies. So this is a quantitative approach for systematically combining results of previous research to arrive at conclusions about the body of research.

That means, it is quantitative (numbers) and is a technique of systematically (methodical), combining (putting together) previous research (what's already done) and bring valid conclusions (new knowledge).

Historical Overview

Ideas behind meta-analysis predate ground work by several decades. Karl Pearson (1904), legendary statistician averaged correlations for studies of the effectiveness of inoculation for typhoid fever. R. A. Fisher (1944) used to say, "When a number of quite independent tests of significance have been made, it sometimes happens that although few or none can be claimed individually as significant, yet the aggregate gives an impression that the probabilities are on the whole lower than would often have been obtained by chance". W. G. Cochran (1953) discussed a method of averaging means across independent studies. He laid-out much of the statistical foundation that modern meta-analysis is built upon (e.g. Inverse variance weighting and homogeneity testing).

Why do Meta-analysis?

Traditional methods of review focus on statistical significance testing but that has several limitations:

a. Highly dependent on sample size

b. Null finding does not carry the same "weight" as a significant finding

   - Significant effect is a strong conclusion

   - Non-significant effect is a weak conclusion. Meta-analysis, on the other hand focuses on the *direction* and *magnitude* of the effects across studies, not statistical significance.

c. This is one of the most important aims of any clinical reader if he/she were to make any useful clinical decisions.

d. Direction and magnitude are represented by the effect size.

Meta-analysis is a common way to draw conclusions in medical research nowadays. This is a quantitative approach for systematically combining results of previous research to arrive at conclusions about the body of research. The characteristic features are given in Tables 32.1, 32.2 and 32.3: Table 32.1 gives general features, while Table 32.2 provides specific features. Table 32.3 gives common summary measures used in meta-analysis.

Since, it is a stepwise inquiry into a well framed question; it starts with identification of studies and ends with statistical analysis of data (Table 32.4).

Table 32.1: Features of meta-analysis

- Quantitative: Numbers
- Systematic: Methodical
- Combining: Putting together
- Previous research: What's already done
- Conclusions: New knowledge

Table 32.2: Details of meta-analysis

- Empirical, rather than theoretical
- Produce quantitative results, rather than qualitative findings
- Examine the same constructs and relationships
- Have findings that can be configured in a comparable statistical form:
  - Effect sizes
  - Correlation coefficients
  - Odds-ratios
  - Proportions
  - Are "comparable" given the question at hand

Table 32.3: Common summary measures used in meta-analysis

- Central tendency research
  - Prevalence rates
- Pre-post contrasts
  - Growth rates
- Group contrasts
  - Experimentally created groups
    - Comparison of outcomes between treatment and comparison groups
  - Naturally occurring groups
    - Comparison of spatial abilities between boys and girls
    - Rates of morbidity among high-and low-risk groups

Table 32. 4: Process of meta-analysis

- Identify your studies
- Determine eligibility of studies
  - Inclusion: Which ones to keep
  - Exclusion: Which ones to throw out
- Abstract data from the studies
- Analyze data in the studies statistically

Importance of Effect Size

Effect size is the minimal measurable difference that can be detected and is clinically or otherwise useful. It would be appropriate to say that the effect size makes meta-analysis possible. It is the "dependent variable" and it standardizes findings across studies such that they can be directly compared.

Any standardized index can be an "effect size" (e.g. standardized mean difference, correlation coefficient, odds-ratio) as long as it meets the following (Table 32.5).

Table 32.5: Effect size in meta-analysis

- It is comparable across studies (generally requires standardization)
- Represents the magnitude and direction of the relationship of interest
- It is independent of sample size
- Different meta-analyses may use different effect size indices

Getting Started

So meta-analysis starts with identification of studies. The process is as given below (Table 32.6). It starts with the inclusion criteria (Table 32.7).

Table 32.6: Process and steps of meta-analysis
- Be methodical: Plan first
- List of popular databases to search
  - Pubmed/medline
  - Embase
  - Cochrane review/trials register
- Other strategies you may adopt
  - Hand search (go to the library...)
  - Personal references, and emails
  - web, e.g. Google (http://scholar.google.com)

Inclusion and Exclusion of Studies

It is critical to have an explicit inclusion and exclusion criteria. The broader the research domain, the more detailed they tend to become. Refine criteria as you interact with the literature (Table 32.7) and then develop inclusion and exclusion criteria (Table 32.8).

Table 32.7: Components of detailed inclusion criteria
- Key variables
- Research methods
- Cultural and linguistic range
- Time frame
- Publication types

Table 32.8: Rejection/exclusion criteria
- Errors in studies (too many confounders/biases)
- Being too restrictive may restrict ability to generalize
- Being too inclusive may weaken the confidence that can be placed in the findings
- Language barrier (often English language studies are included)
- Too short duration studies
- Studies on healthy volunteers alone
- Duplication
- Trials without results

Exclusion Criteria

Some studies will eventually have to be excluded. These may invariably have low qualities. Reasons of rejections are given below (Table 32.9).

Table 32.9: Searching the literature
- Formulate your question appropriately
- If you are searching pubmed
  - Use Medical Subject Headings (MeSH) [1]
  - Lookup word in text word, abstract, title [2]
  - Combine [1] with [2] using boolean logic
  - Set-up proper filters

Since searching the literature is an important component, it is imperative to do it methodically and keep a good record (Table 32.10, Fig. 32.1).

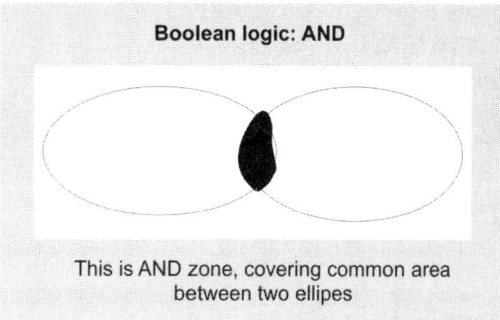

Boolean logic: AND

This is AND zone, covering common area between two ellipses

Fig 32.1: Various key terms can be united by "and". Named after the nineteenth-century mathematician George Boole, Boolean logic is a form of algebra in which all values are reduced to either TRUE or FALSE

Fixed Effect vs Random Effect Model

There are two popular statistical models for meta-analysis, the fixed-effect model and the random-effects model. Under the fixed-effect model we assume that there is one true effect size that underlies all the studies in the analysis, and that all differences in observed effects are due to sampling error. By contrast, under the random-effects model we allow the true effect sizes to differ—it is possible that all studies share a common effect size, but it is also possible that the effect size varies from study to study. Several softwares are available to analysis data in meta-analysis (Table 32.10). Model steps for fixed effect size are given below:

a. Conduct if it is reasonable to assume underlying treatment effect is SAME for all studies (fixed effect).

b. Pooling of data and calculation of odds ratio (OR), e.g. Mantel Haenszel OR.

c. Test of heterogeneity if significant, go for *random effects model.*

d. Short confidence interval (95% CI) for summary

e. Assume that true log odds ratio comes from a normal distribution

f. Method of calculating OR: Der Simonian Lair's method (DSL) of calculating odds' ratio.

Table 32.10: Several softwares are available for meta-analysis

- Free software:
  - EpiMeta: From Epi Info
  - Revman: From Cochrane Collaboration
  - "meta" package in R for statistical computing
- Non-free
  - meta module in STATA

Forest Plot

This is a graphical display of results of clinical trials using a plot where the dotted line passes across null, or 1.0 and the risk estimate of each study is lined up on each side of the dotted line, with 95% CI spread as the line. The diamond on the plot is the summary estimate and the two ends of the diamond indicate 95% confidence interval.

Funnel Plot

Funnel plot depicts the effect size against the sample size of the study. To study a funnel plot, one would have to look at its lower left corner, that's where negative or null studies are located. If funnel plot is empty, this indicates publication bias. Note that here, the plot fits in a funnel, and that the left corner is

not all that empty, but we cannot rule out publication bias (Fig. 32.2).

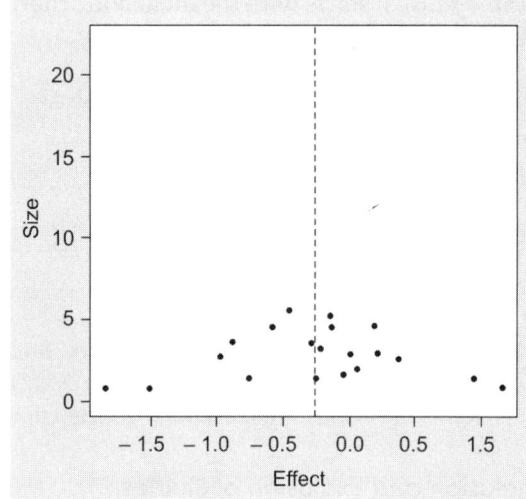

Fig. 32.2: Funnel plot

Strengths

Meta-analyses impose a discipline on the process of summing up research findings. They represent findings in a more differentiated and sophisticated manner than conventional reviews. They are capable of finding relationships across studies that are obscured in other approaches, e.g. systematic reviews and randomized trials and surely in traditional reviews. One of the major strength of meta-analysis is that they protects against over-interpreting differences across studies. Meta-analysis can handle a large numbers of studies as opposed to traditional reviewed. Statistical pooling of data will give results far superior to traditional reviews.

Limitations

We only included published studies because they have been "peer-reviewed" argument. Significant findings are more likely to be published than nonsignificant findings. One should be critical to try to identify and retrieve all studies that meet eligibility criteria be positive or negative. The search strategies should be comprehensive and likely to avoid bias in the studies identified for inclusion. Some other limitations are given in Table 32.11.

Table 32.11: Limitations of meta-analysis

- Meta-analysis require a good deal of effort
- Knowledge of statistics needed
- "Apples and oranges" criticism (studies may be different)
- Most meta-analyses include "blemished" studies to one degree or another (e.g. a randomized design with attrition)
- Analysis of between study differences is fundamentally correlational

Bibliography

1. Introduction to Meta-Analysis Charles DiMaggio, PhD. www.columbia.edu/~cjd11/charles_dimaggio/.../metaAnalysis2011.pdf. (Assessed online 18th March 2016).

2. Meta-analysis fixed effect vs random effects. pdf. https://www.meta-analysis.com/.../Meta-analysis%20fixed%20effect%20. (Assessed online 18th March 2016).

3. What is Boolean Logic? Webopedia. www.webopedia.com/TERM/B/Boolean_logic.html (Assessed online 18th March 2016).

4. What is meta-analysis?-Medical Sciences Division, Oxford. www.medicine.ox.ac.uk/bandolier/painres/download/whatis/meta-an.pdf (Assessed online 18th March 2016).

Design and Execution of Clinical Trials

World Health Organization defines a clinical trial as "any research study that prospectively assigns human participants or groups of humans to one or more health-related interventions to evaluate the effects on health outcomes." Randomization a commonly used term in clinical trial designs refers to the method of assignment of the intervention/comparisons. International Council on Harmonization of technical requirement for use of pharmaceuticals in humans (in short referred as ICH) has adopted "good clinical Practice Guidelines" on 1st May' 1996.

Mostly RCTs are done in medicine rather than surgery. The Clinical Trials Registry of India (CTRI), is a free and online public record system for registration of clinical trials being conducted in India that was launched on 20th July 2007 (www.ctri.nic.in). Initiated as a voluntary measure, since 15th June 2009, trial registration in the CTRI has been made mandatory by the Drugs Controller General of India. The present chapter gives an overview of the process of clinical trials.

Introduction

Clinical trials are considered to be the best tools to assess safety and evaluate the efficacy of clinically administered drugs/therapies/devices/procedures or to compare them with each other.

Clinical trials are systematic scientific experiments and students of medicine/biomedical sciences/clinical research are expected to be conversant with methods of clinical research including their shortfalls, and strengths. Of late, the trend of clinical research

in India has grown and increasing number of medical/biomedical students have keen in interest in clinical research. It is also an integral part of postgraduate curriculum.

What are Clinical Trials?

National Institute of Health, USA defines clinical trials as "biomedical or health related research studies that follow a predefined protocol". It could be of two types: interventional and observational. In the former, any drug or device is tested, while in later, the patients are observed by investigators and health outcome is tested. Trials can be funded by physicians, individuals, organizations, medical institutions, or federal agencies, such as Indian Council of Medical Research in India and National Institute of Health in the US. A trial can take place in medical colleges, institutions, doctors' offices, or community clinics.

Why do Clinical Trials?

Usually, a medicine or a device to be tested is identified and this is followed by one or more pilot trials to gain insight into the design of clinical trial to be followed. Generally, elderly, pregnant women and children are excluded from clinical trials. Therefore, information about the use of drugs in these populations comes from practical use of drugs in clinical settings rather than clinical trials.

Randomized Clinical Trials

In randomized trials, the participants have an equal chance to be assigned to one of two or more groups: One gets the most widely accepted treatment (standard treatment). The other gets the new treatment being tested, which researchers hope and have reason to believe will be better than standard treatment. The clinical trials could be of several types (Fig. 33.1, Table 33.1).

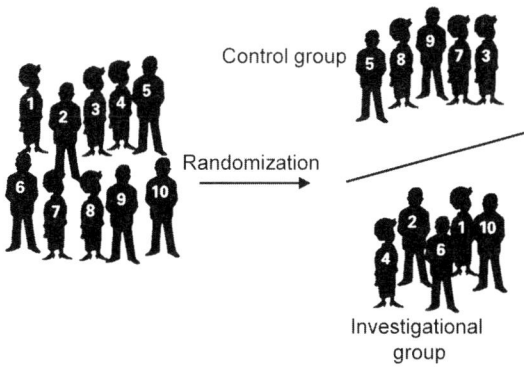

Control group

Randomization

Investigational group

Fig. 33.1: The process of clinical research involves randomization where each groups gets an equal chance of getting selected

Table 33.1: Types of clinical trials

Treatment trials

Diagnostic trials

Screening trials

Quality of life trials

Preventive trials

Compassionate use trials/expanded access

What do Clinical Trials Aim to Achieve?

The purpose of clinical trials is to discover if a drug works and how well if it does. Clinical trials also discover if it has any harmful effects or not. Trials explore the benefit-harm-risk profile of a drug and if it does more good than harm, and how much more? If it has a potential for harm, how probable and how serious is the harm could also be quantified.

In brief, clinical trials do, in general, tell us a good deal about how well a drug works and what potential harm it may cause. Most importantly, they provide information which should be reliable for larger populations with the same characteristics as the trial group-age, gender, state of health, ethnic origin, and so on. However, clinical trials are not infallible. They are conducted in a relatively small number hence, rare side effects may be missed.

Variables in Clinical Trials

The variables in a clinical trial are specified and controlled and the results relate only to the population of which the trial group is a representative sample. A clinical trial can never tell the whole story of the effects of a drug in all situations. A clinical trial must tell about the acceptable balance of benefit and harm. This helps clinicians weigh the information accordingly and take proper decision.

Methodological Issues

Role of clinical trial design and statistical analysis is vital to clinical trials as per ICH guidelines. Methodology starts with submission of a protocol or the procedure document. Students in their study period, deposit thesis protocol for their postgraduate study programs. This is also increasingly getting popular in undergraduate period. In some medical colleges in India faculty members are expected to serve as guide to undergraduate period and students are supposed to submit research projects under their supervision. In others, students do it voluntarily. A protocol will include what is the type of study, what methods adopted, drugs, dosage, monitoring, duration of study.

Investigators could start recruiting the patients and in case he/she is unable to recruit sufficient number; then a trial could be multi-centric. These decisions are generally, settled before hand at the stage of protocol submission.

How to Recruit Patients in Clinical Trials?

Generally, recruitment follows a standard protocol. Advertisements appear in local periodicals or mostly in India, on institute noticeboards. Upon recruitment, patients are asked to attend the research clinic on a given date and time. Protocol is then explained to them in detail.

Before committing, one should evaluate the enrollment criteria to see if they are suitable or not. One has to then develop a recruitment plan and one should be sure that the entire team is committed. Instilling the confidence in research subjects is essential. Table 33.2 below gives the sources where the subjects could be recruited.

Table 33.2: Sources of subjects

- **Chart review:** Pulling patients from the existing schedule of patients: normal patient population
- **Database:** Using a diagnosis code or billing code to pull all patients that match within a certain time frame
- **Referrals:** Some physicians can send out formal letters to PCP or other physicians that might see patients that match inclusion/exclusion
- **Advertising:** Must be approved by IRB: can be google ads, newspapers, radio, etc.

Screening of Subjects

The steps listed below are the industry standard for screening potential subjects like for example, one has to determine medical history, medications the patients are on, test/procedure results, Lab results, etc. also one has to perform physical examination, and perform needed investigations. It is important to know that for wash out period, one would have to withdraw certain medications.

Dropouts

Common reasons for dropouts include: Difficulty complying with the protocol—dosages, timelines, or procedures, etc. or adverse events, loss of motivation, peer pressure, etc. Additional reasons could be financial constraints, disease improvement or lack of improvement, etc. The following could be retention strategies (Table 33.3).

Table 33.3: Retention strategies

1. Maintain communication
2. Listen to the patient
3. Be convenient
4. Maintain a positive attitude
5. Know the protocol

Designing Clinical Trials

Parallel Design

This is a study which is simple one where two treatments are compared. Usually, one is a test therapy while the 2nd is a standard therapy. The allocation of subjects to groups is achieved by randomization. The subjects are the group-I are labeled as treatment group, while in the group-II they are labeled as control group. The number of subjects need not to be the same. The design is commonly chosen in randomized controlled trials. The analysis boils down to a simple t test using a mean or proportion.

Crossover Design

There are two treatments that need to be compared using a crossover study. In such a study, both groups receive each treatment. Randomization is used to determine the order in which they will receive a particular treatment, i.e. whether it will be A followed by B or B followed by A.

Crossover trial reduces the variability between patients because the patients are compared with regard to treatment A and B. Crossover cannot be used if only one form of treatment is being used. Order of treatment may also affect the analysis due to carry over effect.

Factorial Design

This type of design allows investigator to evaluate more than one intervention ion in a single experiment. Whether the treatments are independent or they are complimentary; they can be compared. If we follow a simple example, this is a 2 × 2 design where two treatments are involved at two levels. For example, in a trial involving diabetic patients; patients are randomized to receive low dose aspirin vs placebo and then ticlopidine vs placebo.

Randomization

Since randomization lies at the heart of clinical trials as experimental studies; it is important to explain this here. In clinical trials; groups must be alike in all important aspects and only differ in the intervention each group receives. In practical terms, "comparable treatment groups" means "alike on the average". Each participant has the equal chance of getting any of the treatment under the study.

The allocation is carried out using a chance mechanism so that neither the participant nor the investigator will know which will be assigned to whom. That means the selection of treatment/control group will be made by chance. The purpose of doing this is to minimize bias. Several methods exist for randomization and have been detailed in the appropriate topics. Examples include: Fixed allocation randomization, simple (e.g. flipping a coin), blocked, stratified or adaptive randomization, etc.

Blinding

This is done to avoid any conscious or subconscious influence and allow fair evaluation of the outcomes.

Response Variables

These are variables under study and include drug dose, biologic activity, biomarkers, surrogate outcome, toxicity, etc. Additionally, diagnosis of the patient and final clinical outcome could be response variables.

Placebos

The traditional 'double-blind' randomized control trial uses a placebo to conceal allocation. There are a number of advantages to using a placebo that reduces non-selection bias. A placebo should look or feel and taste the same as the active treatment, which may be difficult. Sham surgery is sometimes used as a 'placebo' surgery. Placebo 'talk' therapy in psychological therapies is another example of placebo. However, placebo to a clinical trial professional means a drug that is used to conceal the real medicine and look like real by itself.

Pitfalls of Randomized Trials

Clinical trials represent the best study design to know about the efficacy of drugs; however, they are not infallible.

Disadvantages of Randomized Trials

1. Generalizable results?
   - Participants studied may not represent general study population.
2. Recruitment
   - Hard
3. Acceptability of randomization process
   - Some physicians will refuse
   - Some participants will refuse
4. Administrative complexity.

Blinding in Clinical Trials

Blinding means concealment. The single blind means the subject do not know what treatment group they have been assigned. The double blind means subject and investigator do not know treatment assignments.

Non-randomized Trials

Early studies of new and untried therapies are usually done without using randomization. Uncontrolled early phase studies where the standard is relatively ineffective could be a good situation to try non-randomized trial.

Sample Size Calculation

Clinical trial is basically the study of an experiment type among people. One would naturally need enough participants to answer the question. Surely, one should not enroll more than needed to answer the question as it could be a waste of available resources. Sample size is an estimate, using guidelines and assumptions.

Inclusion and Exclusion Criteria

All the clinical trials have set guidelines as to who can participate or who could be left out. Factors that allow someone to participate in trials are 'inclusion criteria' and factor, that will disallow are known as 'exclusion criteria'. These could be based upon age, gender, type and stage of disease, previous treatment history, and many other conditions. So a subject must qualify for the study, before joining in. Subjects could be healthy or those who are affected with particular conditions. So, it is imperative that we know what are the criteria that we are following in particular study.

Phases of Clinical Trials

Though, this has been described elsewhere also in this book but for the sake of connection with the content, it has been described here too.

- **Phase I:** First done in healthy subjects for safety analysis and pharmacokinetic considerations.
- **Phase II:** First in patients; dose, dosage form, etc. are decided.
- **Phase III:** Efficacy is studied and adverse drug reactions are noted.
- Post marketing surveillance or Phase IV: Evaluation in the real clinical setting is done via this.

Phase I

- **Objectives**
  - To find out a safe and well-tolerated dose.
  - To see if pharmacokinetics differ much from animal to man so that the dosages can be planned.
  - To see if kinetics show proper absorption, bioavailability to ensure the pharmacokinetic parameters.
  - To detect effects unrelated to the expected action.
  - To detect any predictable toxicity.

- **Inclusion criteria**
  - Healthy volunteers: Uniformity of subjects: age, sex, nutritional status should be there. Also, a written and informed consent a must.
  - Exception: Patients only for toxic drugs, e.g. anti-HIV, anticancer drugs where it would not be appropriate to expose subjects.

- **Exclusion criteria**
  - Women of child bearing age, children, elderly.

- **Methods**
  - First in humans: Small number of healthy volunteers. First done in a small group of 20 to 25. One has to start with a dose

of about 1/10 to 1/5 tolerated animal dose. Slowly the dose is increased to find a safe tolerated dose.

  - If the dose is found to be safe then the same is used in a larger group of up to about 50–75.
  - No blinding is done here and the study is performed by clinical pharmacologists.
  - Centre has emergency care and facility for kinetics study and the study is performed in a single centre. The study takes 3–6 months and has about 70% success rate!

Phase II

This phase is first done in patients and is different from the study done in healthy volunteers. Early phase II studies are done using 20–200 patients with relevant disease/s. Therapeutic benefits and adverse drug reactions are evaluated. One would have to establish a dose range to be used in late phase. It is done single blind (only patient knows) comparison with standard drug.

- Late phase is done in larger number of patients, e.g. 50–500 and is double blind. The drug is compared with a placebo or standard drug.
- Outcomes
  - This study assesses efficacy against a defined therapeutic endpoint. The study notices detailed pharmacokinetic and pharmacodynamic data. This study establishes a dose and a dosage form for future trials.
- This type of study takes 6 months to 2 years and has a 35% success rate.

Phase III

- These are large scale studies done as randomized controlled trials. Target population is usually 250–1000 patients. Usually they are performed by clinicians in the hospital. This type of study minimizes errors of phases I and II.
- **Methods**
  - Usually done multicentric and hence ensure geographic and ethnic variations.

This type of trial design explores different patient subgroups, e.g. pediatric, geriatric, renal impaired, etc.

- Randomized allocation of test drug/placebo/standard drug. It is double blinded and is crossover design.
- Vigilant recording of all adverse drug reactions
- Rigorous statistical evaluation of all clinical data

• **Takes a long time:** Up to 5 years (25% success):

Phase IV

• No fixed duration/patient population
• Starts immediately after marketing
• Report all ADRs
• Helps to detect
  - Rare ADRs
  - Drug interactions
  - Also new uses for drugs (sometimes called Phase V).

Informed Consent

Before a subject decides to participate in the trial, he/she is given full details about the study explaining pros and cons. Note that informed consent is not a contract and patient can withdraw anytime during the course of study. He she is told:

  a. Nature of study
  b. Duration
  c. What dose, what treatment schedule he/she is supposed to follow?
  d. Type of side effects expected are told
  e. Clear instructions should be given when to report to the doctor in case of side effects
  f. Compensation could be offered to the patient in case he/she develops serious side effects. Treatment of complications or side effects arising out of side effects should be done free of cost.

Study Approval

In many countries like the US, every study needs to be approved by Institutional Review Board. In India too, many institutes and medical colleges have ethical committees that meet periodically to discuss the prospective research proposals.

Ethical Committee

The **ethics committee** is an independent body in the institutes/medical colleges and it consists of healthcare professionals and non-medical members, whose responsibility is to protect the rights, safety and well-being of human subjects involved in a clinical trial and to provide them information about the safety and relevance of the same.

Washout

Sometimes, a treatment to be tested may overlap with the existing treatment to be tested. For example, if we are testing a new medicine for patients with a painful disorder of mouth and face (e.g. trigeminal neuralgia); then, we will have to make sure that patients should not have been taking any existing drug known to be effective in same disorder, e.g. carbamazepine/phenytoin. If patients are taking some of these, then, a washout period of 1–2 weeks may be recommended before they are recruited into clinical trials.

Follow-up

This is a standard procedure in which patients are assessed and documented about safety and efficacy of drugs. A detailed assessment of adverse drug reactions is made. It may include interviews, examinations, laboratory tests, adverse event detection/reporting and quality assurance of the products in question.

Data Analysis

This is a critical step. One would have to take into account the occurrence of event, timeline of event, mean level of therapeutic response, duration of response, intention-to-treat, etc. to be able to good data analysis one should know about explanatory variables, subgroups, adjusted vs unadjusted groups and specify in advance the primary and secondary objectives. Statistical approach and package used should be carefully described.

Clinical Trial Protocol

This is a carefully prepared document. Background/justification should be noted. One should clearly specify what does the study add in the light of what is already known about the subject. The protocol should explicitly state hypothesis, study design and methods, types of study, comparison, inclusion and exclusion criteria, description of intervention, concomitant therapy, etc.

The protocol should enlist examination procedures (baseline, follow-up, outcome assessment), intervention assignment procedures, monitoring and management and data and safety monitoring, etc. Adverse event assessment method, reporting, contingency procedures, withdrawal criteria should be mentioned.

Statistics should be described in detail, e.g. sample size, method of calculation of the same, software package for analysis, analysis plans and participant protection issues (including legal framework/compensation, etc).

Conclusions

A Clinical Trials Administrator (CTA) primarily manages the administrative aspects of clinical trials, at every stage of the process starting to end. So the administrators of clinical trials play an essential role in the clinical trial process. Working with protocols (study plans), they prepare, distribute, track and file clinical trial documents. They may also deal with suspected unexpected serious adverse reaction notifications, although in some companies there are specific administrators who work alongside the CTAs for serious adverse events. Most clinical trial administrators work for pharmaceutical companies. They may also work for bio-technology companies, which instead work with biological medicines. CTAs may also work for Contract Research Organisations (CROs). These companies provide a range of services to pharmaceutical organisations wishing to outsource aspects of the research process. Their services include product development, data management and medical writing. The CTAs are office based, and spend the majority of the day working on a computer, using company's own software, therefore computer literacy is essential. They may have to visit a dedicated filing and scanning room when dealing with documents. CTAs work with staff at investigator sites, which are the hospitals that carry out the trial. Because of the ethical issues associated with clinical trials, CTAs must adhere to ICH Good Clinical Practice (GCP) guidelines, which cover all aspects of a trial. These dictate that the results are credible and that the trial subjects are protected. They must also work in accordance with Standard Operating Procedures (SOPs). These are written instructions that dictate how a process must be carried out. Every pharmaceutical company has its own SOPs.

Bibliography

1. Clinical Trial Administrator. https://myjobsearch. com/careers/clinical-trials-administrator.html (Downloaded on April 15th 2017).
2. Design, execution, and management of medical device clinical trials. http://onlinelibrary.wiley. com/doi/10.1002/9780470475911. fmatter/ pdf (Downloaded on May4th 2017).
3. Understanding clinical trials. http://clinicaltrials. gov/ct2/info/understand (Accessed on May' 2016).

Systematic Review

Learning objectives

Systematic reviews are undertaking of a review with a focused research question that tries to identify, appraise, select and synthesize all high quality research evidence relevant to that question. In summary, systematic reviews are publication subtypes aimed to draw conclusions from the wide body of evidence available. Randomized Clinical Trials (RCTs) are considered to be the gold standard methods of evaluation of scientific information in medical world; however, the systematic reviews synthesize information from large number of RCTs. Systematic reviews can help us make a decision about safety, efficacy and tolerability of drugs.

Introduction

A systematic review is a multistage process aimed to identify all available and reliable publications regarding a specific problem, to evaluate their reliability and to compile available data in a quantitative (meta-analysis) or qualitative manner. It should be noted that the traditional reviews differ from the systematic reviews (Table 34.1). Systematic reviews should have the following qualities (Box 34.1).

Box 34.1: Qualities of a good systematic review

- A clearly defined, explicit question.
- A comprehensive and systematic search for studies.
- An explicit, reproducible strategy for screening and including studies
- Explicit, reproducible data extraction (coding)
- Appropriate analysis and reporting of results
- Interpretations supported by data
- Implications for future research, and if relevant, for policy or practice.

Table 34.1: Features of traditional reviews and systematic reviews

Traditional reviews	Systematic review
• Narrative writing	• Starts with a proper research question or hypothesis.
• Tries to draw inferences based upon published studies	• Well-defined inclusion and exclusion criteria is needed.
• Lack of statistical intervention	
• Proper protocol formation is not needed.	
– Inclusion and exclusion is not needed.	
– No clear hypothesis or research question	
• Key words not very important except for listing purpose in data bases.	• Key words define the search and will be selected as per the review question.
• Less reliable; though widely read by students,	• Highly reliable.
• Quality of studies is not given much of preference.	• Quality of studies is given much of preference.
• Subjectivity may come in; bias prone.	• Subjectivity very less lively.
• Help in evidence-based medicine.	• Very helpful in evidence-based medicine; in formulation of guidelines.

(Contd...)

Table 34.1: Features of traditional reviews and systematic reviews *(Contd...)*

Traditional reviews	Systematic review
• Broad in scope	• Focused.
• Qualitative summary	• Qualitative and quality,
• Less critical	• Critical analysis
• Not based upon software	• Analysis based on software

Table 34.2: Need of systematic reviews

• To get new evidence for patient management.
• Avoid implementation that can harm patient.
• To get updated knowledge about disease and its features.
• To generate new modules for clinical training.
• To keep practitioners up-to-date about evidence based medicine.

The Importance of Systematic Literature Reviews

Most research starts with a literature review of some sort. However, unless a literature review is thorough and fair, it is of little scientific value. This is the main rationale for undertaking systematic reviews. A systematic review synthesizes existing work in a manner that is fair and seen to be fair. For example, systematic reviews must be undertaken in accordance with a predefined search strategy. The search strategy must allow the completeness of the search to be assessed. In particular, researchers performing a systematic review must make every effort to identify and report research that does not support their preferred research hypothesis as well as identifying and reporting research that supports it. Systematic reviews are needed for several reasons (Table 34.2).

Why do Systematic Reviews?

The need for a systematic review arises from the requirement of researchers to summarize all existing information about some phenomenon in a thorough and unbiased manner. This may be in order to draw more general conclusions about some phenomenon than is possible from individual studies, or may be undertaken as a prelude to further research activities.

Advantages and Disadvantages (Fig. 34.1)

The advantages of systematic literature reviews are that: Systematic reviews are well-defined methodology makes it less likely that the results of the literature are biased, although it does not protect against publication bias in the

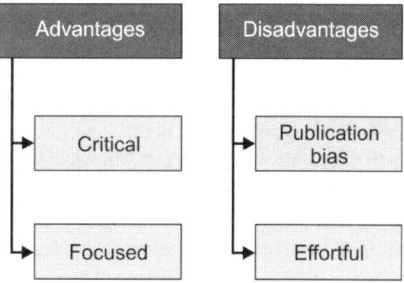

Fig. 34.1: The process of systematic reviews can be tedious and can be difficult to manage. In the process, one will have to define the question, develop the hypothesis, have clear inclusion and exclusion criteria, stick to the particular keywords, and then search the items thoroughly. Help of software or that of the statistician may be needed. However, the results can be rewarding. It should be known that the publication bias is very less likely but systematic reviews do not protect against the publication bias totally

primary studies. Systematic reviews can provide information about the effects of some phenomenon across a wide range of settings and empirical methods. If studies give consistent results, systematic reviews provide evidence that the phenomenon is robust and transferable. If the studies give inconsistent results, sources of variation can be studied.

In the case of quantitative studies, it is possible to combine data using meta-analytic techniques. This increases the likelihood of detecting real effects that individual smaller studies are unable to detect.

The major disadvantage of systematic literature reviews is that they require considerably more effort than traditional literature reviews. In addition, increased power for meta-analysis can also be a disadvantage, since it is possible to detect small biases as well as true effects.

Features of Systematic Literature Reviews

Some of the features that differentiate a systematic review from a conventional expert literature review are:

a. Systematic reviews start by defining a review protocol that specifies the research question being addressed and the methods that will be used to perform the review.

b. Systematic reviews are based on a defined search strategy that aims to detect as much of the relevant literature as is possible.

c. Systematic reviews document their search strategy so that readers can assess their rigour and the completeness and repeatability of the process (bearing in mind that searches of digital libraries are almost impossible to replicate).

d. Systematic reviews require explicit inclusion and exclusion criteria to assess each potential primary study.

e. Systematic reviews specify the information to be obtained from each primary study including quality criteria by which to evaluate each primary study.

f. A systematic review is a prerequisite for quantitative meta-analysis.

Systematic reviews though are time taking, but are rewarding and are done for several reasons (Table 34.3).

The literature Review Process

A systematic literature review involves several discrete activities. Existing guidelines for systematic reviews have slightly different

Table 34.3: Critical features of systematic reviews

- Support evidence-based practice in medicine
- Research
- Generate clinical policies or guidelines
- Stimulate publications
- Personal professional development and training

suggestions about the number and order of activities. However, the medical guidelines and sociological textbooks are broadly in agreement about the major stages in the process.

The Steps in a Systematic Review

Since systematic reviews are tedious and need to be done methodically, one would have to follow the steps (Table 34.4, Fig. 34.2).

Table 34.4: Broad steps of performing systematic reviews

- Formulate clear clinical questions from our knowledge needs
- Search the literature to identify relevant articles
- Critically appraise the evidence for its validity and usefulness
- Synthesize usable clinical evidence

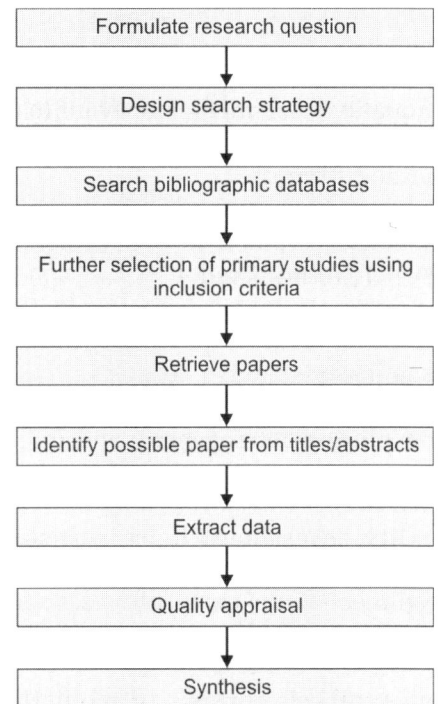

Fig. 34.2: Stepwise approach towards conducting systematic reviews. The process starts with formulation of research question and synthesis of information from available literature

Step 1: Framing of the Questions for a Review

- Clear, unambiguous and structured questions before beginning the systematic review work to be addressed should be specified.
- Once the systematic review questions have been set, modifications to the protocol should be allowed only if alternative ways of defining the populations, interventions, outcomes or study designs become apparent.

Step 2: Identifying Relevant Work

- The search for studies should be extensive using multiple data base.
- Multiple resources (both computerized and printed) should be searched without language restrictions.
- The study selection criteria should flow directly from the review questions and be specified *a priori.*
- Reasons for inclusion and exclusion should be specified and should be strict.

Step 3: Assessing the Quality of Studies

Study quality assessment is relevant to every step of a review.

- Question formulation.
- Study selection criteria should describe the minimum acceptable level of design.
- Selected studies should be subjected to a more refined quality assessment by the use of general critical appraisal guides and design-based quality checklists.
- Detailed quality assessments will be used for exploring heterogeneity and informed decisions regarding suitability of meta-analysis.
- Quality assessment help in assessing the strength of inferences and making recommendations for future research.

Step 4: Summarizing the Evidence

- Data synthesis consists of tabulation of study characteristics, quality and effects as well as use of statistical methods for exploring differences between studies and combining their effects (meta-analysis).
- Exploration of heterogeneity and its sources should be planned in advance.

Step 5: Interpreting the Findings

- The processes highlighted in each of the four steps above should be met. The risk of publication bias and related biases should be explored before concluding.
- Exploration for heterogeneity should help determine whether the overall summary can be trusted, and, if not, the effects observed in high-quality studies should be used for generating inferences.
- Any recommendations should be graded by reference to the strengths and weaknesses of the evidence.

Summary

Compared to traditional reviews, systematic reviews use a more systematic approach to data collection, and have more transparent and explicit procedures. Thus systematic reviews have less potential for hidden assumptions or biases to drive results. Systematic reviews focus on the magnitude of effects rather than statistical significance. Hence, the results of systematic reviews end in conclusions that are less bound by context than conclusions that arise from individual studies.

Bibliography

1. Guidelines for performing Systematic Literature Reviews in Software Engineering. http://userpages.uni-koblenz.de/~laemmel/esecourse/slides/slr.pdf (Downloaded on 18th March, 2016).
2. Introduction to Systematic Reviewing and Meta-Analysis. http://www.campbellcollaboration.org/artman2/uploads/1/Valentine_Introduction_Systematic_Reviewing_1.pdf (Downloaded on 18th March, 2016).
3. Khalid S Khan, Regina Kunz, Jos Kleijnen, Gerd Antes, Five steps to conducting a systematic review. J R Soc Med. 2003 Mar; 96(3): 118–121.

Double Blind Randomized Clinical Trials

Learning objectives

Randomized clinical trials are research studies that are aimed to test how well a drug or a medical device or a treatment regiment works in patients. These are aimed to find ways to prevent or treat diseases. One of the most important aims of clinical trials is to compare the different treatments.

Main strengths of clinical trials include best measure of causal relationships, and best design for controlling bias in medical research. They can also be very useful in measuring multiple outcomes at same time. Main weaknesses are high costs, ethical issues may be a problem and compliance may hinder the progress as well.

Introduction

Randomized trials are considered to be the highest form of evidence-accepted in modern times for the safety and efficacy of drug treatment using human subjects. Understanding trials will enable us to be aware of foundations of evidence-based methods in a detailed manner.

A clinical trial is an experiment involving human beings that is designed to evaluate the drugs and to compare their efficacy.

Clinical trial uses placebo or the active drug as a comparator and gives a confirm or refute the claim that the said drug is more effective than the standard drug. The pros and cons are given in Table 35.1.

What is a Control?

In clinical trials, every experiment should have a "control group." People in control group are

Table 35.1: Advantages and disadvantages of randomized controlled clinical trials

Advantages	Disadvantages
• This type of design is good for removing bias	The trial design is expensive
• Blinding and masking is possible and is easy	The participants may not be fully representative of the population
Results can be analyzed using statistical tools.	Loss to follow up can occur
• Generate highest form of evidence that can be imbibed into clinical practice	

treated exactly the same way as the other people in the experiment, except they do not get the "active treatment (e.g. drug)." A "placebo group" is a special kind of control group.

Blinding

This is a form of experiment in which participants are deliberately kept in darkness about whether the patient is taking placebo or the active drug. What is the patients know that what are they taking? It will be difficult for them to exhibit true pharmacological response. It is always going to be mixed with psychological response. Knowing that a patient is getting the placebo can change the way a patient behaves in an experiment. This is called Hawthorne effect. To avoid this effect, blinding is used. A person who is not directly connected with the trial (say a nurse or a pharmacist), will be given the task of assigning random numbers to patients and assign them into two groups, e.g. containing placebo or active comparator as per the protocol.

Blinding therefore ensures that the psychological bias is removed. Also other forms of biases that get eliminated include: observer bias.

For example, if the physician know that he or she has some patients who are "favourite" to him or her; he or she willingly or unknowingly may assign them active "drug". External validity of such a trial is limited.

So, it is clear until and unless there is a comparator, i.e. placebo or the active drug, it is hard to say that the said effect in a clinical trial is due to presence of the drug itself and not due to other factors.

Different Types of Clinical Trials

There are many types of clinical trials but there are four main phases of trials. These include:

Phase I: This is called pharmacokinetic trials. Normally we take 20–50 subjects and try to determine maximally tolerated dose in this form. Safety data gets generated by this type of trial. Nowadays, there is a trend of using pharmacokinetic/pharmacodynamic data (PK/PD) data and make more sense about the way a drug works. Comparator or placebo will not be needed here as we are not trying to test the efficacy (Table 35.2).

Table 35.2: Salient features of phase I studies

- Population:
  - If healthy volunteers—where will you recruit?
  - If ill population—what is standard of care?
- Visit duration:
  - What study personnel need to be available and for how long at each study visit?
  - Where do you have the space to conduct a long visit?
- Design
  - Open label
- Aim
  - Safety

Phase II: This is called efficacy trial. We take around 50–300 patients. We do not take subjects in this form of clinical trial. Our aim is to further confirm findings of the phase I trial and to know what happens when the same results are repeated in a large number of cases (Table 35.3).

Table 35.3: Salient features of phase II studies

- Population
  - Criteria is generally strict—do we have the population?
  - Do we have conflicting studies?
- Duration
  - Studies generally are not long, so when does enrollment end?
  - If subjects have to go off their meds for a period of time, will you expect a high dropout rate?
- Design
  - Randomized—who will randomize subjects?
  - Double blind studies—who is going to be available to unblind if necessary?
- Aim
  - Continued safety evaluations
  - Initial efficacy data

Phase III: This is called randomized trials. Normally, we take 300–100 patients. Since there are a large number of patient intakes, this has to be a highly organized process. Randomization is the cornerstone. Failing of proper randomization will limit the generalizability of trial. It has placebo or active control and we look for the evidence of refuting null hypothesis and accept alternative hypothesis (Table 35.4).

Phase IV: This is pharmacovigilance and is a common type of pragmatic trial. In this form, we try to observe a drug for possible side effects associated with the drug. Since some side effects are always going to be missed if we take a small sample size, our aim is always to take a large sample. Usually it is done in a sample size >1000. Since, it is done after the drug has gotten the final approval for marketing; it is also called phase IV trial or post-marketing surveillance (Table 35.5).

Table 35.4: Salient features of phase III studies

- Population
  - Generally large # of subjects, do we have the capacity to see them?
  - Representative population (broader inclusion/exclusion criteria), do we have these subjects in our clinic?
- Duration
  - Parallels expected treatment use (several days to years)—do we have the capacity to follow the subjects for a long-time?
- Design
  - Generally double bind
- Aims
  - Establish safety and efficacy in the target population

Table 35.5: Salient features of phase IV studies

- Population
  - Population prescribed the drug—who will pay for the drug?
- Duration
  - Long-term for chronic diseases—do we have the capacity to see the subjects for years?
- Design
  - Generally open label
  - Procedures generally same as clinical care—what is research and what is standard of care? Who pays?
- Aim
  - Economic comparisons
  - Quality of life
  - Adherence and compliance

Pharmacologists and pharmacists call it, 'adverse drug reaction monitoring' trial. This is one of the most potent tool to ensure the good drug safety. Case reports by clinicians could be the beginning of some through clinical studies that could be initiated once we get some hint that the drug is associated with side effect/s. This process is known as **signal generation.**

A decision to continue with the drug or to withdraw could be taken based upon the results of phase IV studies. They could also be initiated if we get hints that a already marketed drug for a long-time is associated with a particular side effect. This happened with nimesulide and it was found that the drug was associated with high frequency of hepatic dysfunction in children. A decision of banning the drug in India was taken. So that means, it can be an academic activity that is routinely done in reaching institutions or alternatively a systemic inquiry if adequate signals are generated. True signals however need to be differentiated from false signals. This process is known as **'signal-to-noise'** ratio.

Trial Designs

There are several ways to classify the trial designs:

a. *Parallel group design*: Patients are randomized either to the treatment arm or to the placebo arm or to the (test) and (control) arm using a standard comparators. They are followed up prospectively to know the efficacy difference as and when they emerge. There could be several variants of these:
   - Sequential crossover: A single patient given placebo and continues taking it and later on gets the drug.
   - Group sequential trials: At certain stages that are defined in the protocol; one could get an idea about efficacy of clinical trials. They could be evaluated and stopped when desired results are obtained.
   - Adapted designs: A trial is stopped midway and some changes in design and protocol could be done.

b. *Factorial design*: Normally, patients are assigned one treatment-comparison group and are followed up. In such trial, a single patient may be randomized in two or more groups.

c. *Cluster randomized trial*: This is parallel group design, the only difference is that rather than the individuals being randomized cluster of patients, e.g. hospitals, clinics, or groups of patients are randomized.

Centers

Trials could conveniently be done at a single center. However, nowadays, they are preferably done at multiple centers. Multi centric studies are done for the following reasons:

a. To sufficient number of cases could be found if more than 1 centers are inducted at the same time.

b. To improve generalizability.

Exploratory vs Confirmatory Trial

If we are the first one to conduct a clinical trial, then it is called exploratory trial. Others will have to confirm the results and hence will be called confirmatory trial.

Biases

A clinical trial may or not show the true difference and hence, may be subjected to lot of biases. So, it may have false positive and false negative results. Both biases and contamination cab result. There is a possibility of random error also.

There are two main kind of errors noted in clinical trials:

a. Systematic error

b. Random error

Systematic Error

This can result from the trial design and hence will affect interpretation of results. Mostly, it is related to selection of subjects and outcome measurements. For example, if the investigators know what is being given to which group, they may have a psychological bias and may favour treatment.

Likewise, exclusion of missing subjects due to lack of proper data or compliance may also affect the analysis and interfere with trial results. This may overestimate the benefit offered by the trial. Advanced trial designs seek to eliminate these biases from clinical trials.

Confounding

This is a special form of distorted relationship that may come due to an extraneous variable and we may false attribute it to some other variable. For example, if we wish to know what is the relationship between physical inactivity and heart disease, then a number of potential confounders will come. These include smoking, alcohol, weight, sex, age and hyperlipidemia and diabetes, etc.

How to Deal with Confounding Factors?

Most effective method to deal with con-founders is to randomize the subjects so that they are distributed equally among both groups. Both known and unknown con-founders could be distributed like this.

For example, if age acts as a potential confounder; then stratifying groups into males and females may help. This is known as stratified randomization. Regression and stratified analysis might help to analyze these results during analytic stage.

Random Error

Even in the best of trial design, errors due to measurements, due to individual variations and sampling can occur (MIS). Proper recording of data therefore may be of value. Most studies will be studying only a part of the sample; therefore, one should keep the possibility of sampling error.

How to Deal with Random Error?

This may be reduced by selecting a large number of participants or using special techniques for analysis, e.g. meta-analysis. These are called "studies of studies".

Statistical techniques dealing with such techniques will give an estimate of how likely is it, that the treatment effect reflects the true effect and not otherwise.

Statistical techniques rest on the grounds that there is no statistically significant difference between the two groups (null hypothesis). We wish to reject the null hypothesis at a preset level, called level of significance or alpha level. *P-value* is the probability of rejecting null hypothesis at given level of significance. Smaller is *p-value*, greater is the probability of null hypothesis being untrue or it can be rejected safely. Alpha-level is usually set at 5% level, though it could be set at 1% as well. For behavioral studies, it could be set even at 10% level. Setting it above 10% will give wide error margins unless the sample size is extremely large. At 5% level of significance, we accept that we may be wrong in 1:20 times, and this is called Type I error (alpha-error). Likewise, if there was a true difference but we could not spot it; then it is called Type II error (beta-error).

Usually we summarize the results for an outcome in the form of point estimates such as means or proportions and measures of precision such as confidence interval. A narrow confidence interval means results are more precise. Likewise, a wide confidence interval means results are imprecise.

A 95% confidence interval for the treatment difference will be a range that could present for the treatment effect when calculated 95 out of 100 hypothetical trials.

Testing several hypothesis with clinical trials will always be difficult. Ideally, it should be restricted to one at a time.

Differences between treatments during interim analysis multiple times could lead to an error as well if it is not backed by hypothesis.

Interim Monitoring

Safety of the patients in clinical trials is paramount and hence during interim analysis, attempt is made to monitor safety of drugs in a periodic manner. Safety monitoring board, ethics committees and Drug Controller General of India will ensure that the drug safety data is properly generated. Likewise, if there is major evidence that the desired results have been obtained; then one could stop the trial (stop trial for efficacy).

Final Data Analysis

If there are lots of missing values and also there are issues about the compliance; it may be advisable to do intention-to-treat analysis.

Intention-to-treat analysis deals with outcomes of the patients who were randomized but subsequently discontinued or changed treatment. This is a pragmatic realization of trial and it is taken "as if the patients who were enrolled and randomized, finished trial" as well.

Doing intention-to-treat analysis and using two sided *p-value* is a good fallback options for clinical trials. Moreover, results could be stratified to reduce random error. Time to event end points could be demonstrated by Kaplan-Meier plots. Size of treatment effect could be calculated from Hazard ratios derived from proportional hazard model. Cox regression model could be used to adjust hazard ratio for other factors that might affect prognosis.

Sample size calculations too are detailed right in beginning so as to ensure accuracy. It is important to note that sample size calculations are best done using primary outcome measure. Secondary objectives do not features in the same.

Statistical analysis is pre-specified in protocol and one should preferably stick to the same.

Subgroup analysis could be done using test for heterogeneity to assess for possible interaction effect between treatment and baseline variables.

Consolidated Standards of Reporting Trials (Consort Guidelines)

A trial is published in accordance with statement and guidelines of reporting.

Trial Profile

A trial profile is provided in the clinical trial to describe the flow of participants through each stage of the randomized controlled trial, i.e. enrollment, randomization, treatment allocation, follow-up, etc. Analysis of a clinical trial should be specified and it should also be mentioned if mid-term analysis will be done and if so then at what stage.

The baseline characteristics of patient's, e.g.
• Demographic information
• History of inter-current illnesses, e.g. heart disease/risk factors

- Medical history
- Treatment history

Randomized patients should be comparable as to reduce systematic error.

Conclusions

Randomized clinical trials are the gold standard of efficacy of a clinical trial. Some treatments historically have been used without clinical trials as their evidence has been considered to be "sufficient". Nowadays, however, a new treatment needs to be evaluated in new night. Attempt should be made to deal with major type of errors that may creep during clinical trials, e.g. systematic and random error. We should know, how to deal with those error. Many errors will affect our ability to draw valid conclusions.

The main types of errors that can arise and can seriously compromise our ability to draw valid conclusions from clinical trials (external validity). So, we should minimize bias and maximize precision (i.e. have a narrow confidence interval). A clear definition of primary and secondary objectives has to be there. Selection of subjects, i.e. inclusion and exclusion criteria should be such that it minimizes systematic error. Potential errors or confounders could be dealt by matching and randomization so that potential confounders are distributed evenly among groups.

Finally, the trial should be ethically sound and answers a question: "is the new treatment similar, better or worse than placebo? Safety monitoring during trials is important and so is interim analysis. If the trial has achieved its desired end point; then one can stop it for efficacy.

Bibliography

1. Clinical trials. https://medlineplus.gov/clinicaltrials.html (Downloaded on May 4th 2017).
2. Controlled and uncontrolled studies. https://faculty.unlv.edu/beisecker/Courses/Phi-102/Controlled_Studies.htm (Downloaded on April 17th 2017).
3. Overview of clinical trials. http://www.centerwatch.com/clinical-trials/overview.aspx (Downloaded on May 4th 2017).
4. Randomized control trial. https://himmelfarb.gwu.edu/tutorials/studydesign101/rcts.html (Downloaded on April 17th 2017).

Interpreting Research Data

Learning objectives

Data are distinct pieces of research information. Research data is data that is collected, observed, or created, for purposes of analysis to produce original research results. The word "data" is used throughout this book to refer to research data. Research data can be generated for different purposes and through different processes, and can be divided into different categories. Research data is recorded factual material commonly retained by and accepted in the scientific community as necessary to validate research findings; although the majority of such data is created in digital format, all research data is included irrespective of the format in which it is created.

Introduction

Researchers involved in biomedical research should analyze and interpret their researchers clearly and coherently, as to draw valid conclusion from the data that they have. The researchers should use appropriate statistical tests to make sure that the conclusions that they are making are understood easily by the students and doctors alike.

Mean

Mean is the most commonly used method to describe the data. However, it is useful only when the data follows normal distribution. Otherwise, median may be a better method to explain the same. Standard deviations should be given along with the mean. However, if the range is given it may indicate a good amount of variability in the given data.

Graphs

Graphs are a very popular way of explaining things. The researchers should be careful in explaining the x and y axis. This will give a good deal of idea about the relationships. However, mistakes in explaining the same can distort the values and give a bad idea.

p-value

p-value is the most common way in which the statistical significance of a research data is described. However, it should be borne clearly in mind that whatever is statistically significant, may not always turn out to be clinically significant.

For example, the group means of two groups of dementias with mean MMSE scores of 24 and 25.5 may come out to be statistically significant but may not have value significant value in terms of their clinical significance.

It is also important to know if the *p-values* given are the *p-values* which are one tailed or two tailed. The latter are better.

Bias

It is hard to find studies that are totally free from all kind of biases. Therefore, bias will have to be understood. Bias is a systematic error that creeps into the study and will distort the results. The effect of the bias is usually interpreted as "something that would involve, like is not being compared with like". The following can protect against the bias:

a. Choose the most appropriate design so that the bias can be eliminated at an early stage.

b. Be aware of 'selection' bias when you select subjects for your study. Once the study is done, then the 'measurement bias' will have to be guarded against.

c. 'Response bias' is another type of problem that comes your way, and this can affect the results significantly.

Confounding

Suppose if you want to conclude, that being in air-conditioned office of Dr. Ram Manohar Lohia hospital 8 hours a day will lower your levels of vitamin D and if you ignore the vitamin D intake of your subjects; then the conclusion drawn may be wrong. That means, confounders are "other things" that will affect the results and conclusions. The following two terms should be understood when we analyze the data:

a. **Crude rates:** These are used when the results have not been adjusted as per the confounders.

b. **Adjusted rates:** These are used when the results have not been adjusted as per the confounders. This type of data has undergone statistical transformation for the adjustment of confounders.

Causation in Clinical Research

Over 150 years back, Robert Koch introduced the term causality in clinical medicine by the following criteria:

a. Organism must be associated with the disease.

b. Must be isolated from the diseased organs or patients and be grown in culture.

c. Once inoculated in healthy animals, it must produce the specific disease.

d. It must be recovered from the infected tissues.

Chance, bias or confounding can give a false association and must be guarded against. The criteria were later modified by Bradford Hill and are very popular in clinical research and epidemiological studies. The criteria are as follows:

1. The organism should be consistently associated with the disease.

2. Observed evidence must be consistent.

3. Relationship must be specific.

4. It must be temporal.

5. Gradient should be in favor of causation.

6. Biologically plausible explanation should be there.

7. Coherent evidence should be there.

8. It should be verifiable by experiment.

9. Reasoning should be thereby analogy.

Interpreting Effects

In a hypothetical study, aspirin 75 mg appeared to reduce the risk of myocardial infarction in men by 50%. However, the overall mortality remained unchanged after 2 years of follow-up and there was a trend towards bleeding as side effects due to aspirin. So interpreting this study could be difficult if one would just see at one end point, i.e. the bleeding. The risk reduction is significant and should be interpreted with a pinch of salt as in there are safety issues.

Surrogate Marker

If the surrogate marker has both sensitivity and specificity; then its positive and negative predictive values can be known. The stage is set for the use of this parameter as a surrogate marker. Some of the examples are given below (Table 36.1).

Risks

While interpreting results of studies, it is important to understand the concept of risk. This is because, unless interpreted properly, this can lead to misinformation and miscommunication. A variety of risks need to be understood (Table 36.2).

Table 36.1: Examples of surrogate markers in clinical research

Cardiovascular	Lp (a)
Neurological	Hippocampal volume
Psychiatric	Amygdala volume
Gastroenterology	Liver enzymes
Hematology	CD_4 cell counts
Nephropathy	Serum creatinine/urea

Table 36.2: Concepts of risks

- Basic risk
- Relative risk
- Attributable risk (AR)
- Number needed to treat (NNT)
- Number needed to harm (NNH)
- Risk versus benefit

Relative Risk

This is the incidence of outcome in the exposed group compared to the unexposed group. In statistics and epidemiology, relative risk or risk ratio (RR) is the ratio of probability of an even occurring (e.g. lung cancer) among the exposed groups (e.g. among smokers) compared to unexposed group (e.g. non smokers.

	Outcome	No outcome
Exposed	a	b
Unexposed	c	d

$$\text{Relative} = \frac{\text{Incidence in exposed}}{\text{Incidence in unexposed}} = \frac{a/a+b}{c/c+d}$$

Odds Ratio

Odds ratio (OR) is a measure of association between an exposure and the outcome. OR represents the odds that an outcome will occur given a particular exposure exits (e.g. smoking), compared to odds of the outcome in the absence of the exposure (e.g. no smoking).

$$\text{Odds ratio} = \frac{\text{Odds that the diseased were exposed}}{\text{Odds the controls were exposed}}$$

In epidemiological terms, it would define the odd of having the risk factor in the diseased group compared to those who do not have the disease.

Confidence Interval

It the RR has been reported without giving the confidence interval then the interpretation cannot be done properly. A RR of 1 means, there is no association between the risk factor and the disease. A relative risk may be higher than 1 but it has to be statistically significant.

Attributable Risk and Absolute Risk Reduction (Table 36.3)

Any interpretation of attributable risk thinking based upon just the relative risk could be risky. The only difference between absolute and relative risk is that in the probability of disease is going down due to a treatment and in absolute risk reduction, the probability is going up due to an exposure or risk factor (Table 36.4). Both Number Needed to Treat and Number Needed to Harm are 1 divided by the absolute risk reduction or attributable risk (whichever is more appropriate).

One has to take the disease prevalence into account as well.

Table 36.3: Attributable risk (AR) and absolute risk reduction (ARR)

Attributable risk (AR)	Absolute risk reduction (ARR)
• Probability of disease among those without treatment compared to those who have been treated	• Probability of disease among those who are exposed, e.g. lung cancer among those who smoke compared to lung cancer among those who do not smoke
• Can help in estimating number needed to treat/harm	• Can help in estimating number needed to treat/harm

Ultimate decision about using the drug or withholding the drug treatment will have to be made taking risk versus benefit into account.

Table 36.4: Relative risk and absolute risk

Relative risk (RR)	Absolute risk (AR)
• Measures magnitude of the effect of an intervention • Not very important from a clinical standpoint • Compares two different groups	Clinically important as it would tell how many individuals would actually benefit. It measures the risk of disease overtime, e.g. risk of heart disease, diabetes, etc.

Sensitivity

This is the probability of finding the individuals who have the disease. If the sensitivity of a diagnostic test is high, then the test will have a very low false negatives.

Specificity

This is the ability of a diagnostic test to pick up healthy people. A high specificity would mean, there will be very low false positives in the diagnostic test.

Positive Predictive Value

Given the diagnostic test is positive, what is the chance that the disease is also there. This is because a test may be false positive also.

Number Needed to Treat and Number Needed to Harm Calculation

Both of the important parameters can be calculated as follows:

$$\text{Number needed to treat} = \frac{1}{\text{Absolute risk Reduction}}$$

$$\text{Number needed to harm} = \frac{1}{\text{Attributable risk}}$$

Efficiency of a Diagnostic Test

This is the overall ability of a diagnostic test to classify patients correctly. It can be calculated by adding true positives and true negatives and dividing that with total number of patients.

Interpreting Sensitivity and Specificity

Diagnostic tests are not perfect and increasing the sensitivity will often lead to decreased specificity and *vice versa*. So there has to be a balance maintained between the two. Prevalence is an important determinant to. A small number of false positive cases can be magnified if the disease is rare. So positive predictive value is influenced by a great deal by the disease prevalence too.

Receiver Operator Curve (ROC)

These curves are useful in getting the cut-off for the screening test. Sensitivity can be plotted on vertical axis and a value on the horizontal axis which is calculated by subtracting 1-specificity (Fig. 36.1).

Interpret the Results of Trials

One should be cautious in interpreting the results of uncontrolled trials as there no comparison available. Therefore, drawing inference would be difficult.

Controlled trials are easier to interpret if there is a comparison available with an active comparator. Even if the drug was compared against the placebo, it can suggest that the drug is working. Still the overall conclusion should be made keeping about Safety, Tolerability, Efficacy and Price (STEP) of the drug.

Even if the trial has reported a statistically significant result, it may not be clinically significant.

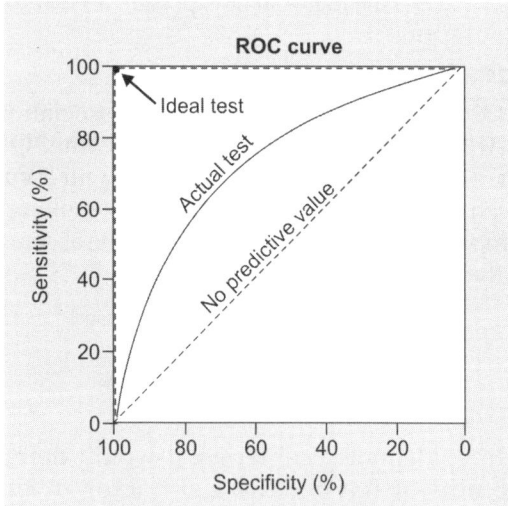

Fig. 36.1: Receiver operating characteristic curve or also called ROC curve is a plot of true positives (those with disease) against false positive (those who do not have the disease) for the different cut-off points of a diagnostic test. That means, it is a reciprocal curve of sensitivity and specificity; any increase in sensitivity will be accompanied by a decrease in specificity (curve movements towards left hand side indicates the curve is closer to the 100% sensitivity indicating its ability to detect the disease)

Interpreting Qualitative Research

One should look for the following:

Credibility means, the explanations offered are logical and could account for the data that is being shown Table 36.5. One should act as "devil's advocate" here and see all possible explanation that could be used to explain the data.

Table 36.5: Important things in qualitative research
- Credibility
- Dependability
- Conformability
- Transferability

Dependability is if the similar data can be reproduced by doing another study. *Conformability* means if the other investigators have the accesses to the data and they can do their own analysis. *Transferability* is the ability to generalize results to larger or different populations.

Conclusions

Data analysis is an attempt by the researcher to summarize collected data. However, interpretation is an attempt to find meaning.

It is important to know that the analysis not left until the end. To avoid collecting data that are not important the researcher must ask: How am I going to make sense of this data? And as they collect data the researcher must ask:
- What and why is participant's response/s?
- What does this focus mean?
- What else do we want to know?
- What new ideas have emerged?
- Is this new information?

The assembly of this information can lead to good interpretation and future recommendations.

Bibliography

1. Data analysis and interpretation. www.uio.no/ studier/emner/matnat/ifi/INF4260/h10/.../ DataAnalysis.pdf (Downloaded on July5th, 2017)

2. Data management. https://blogs.ucl.ac.uk/ rdm/2015/09/what-is-research-data/ (Downloaded on April 17th 2017).

3. Research data. http://www2.le.ac.uk/services/ research-data/rdm/what-is-rdm/research-data (Downloaded on April 17th 2017).

4. What is research data? https://www.bu.edu/ datamanagement/background/whatisdata/ (Downloaded on April 17th 2017).

Chapter

37

Publishing a Research Paper

Learning objectives

One would have to familiarize oneself with publication process. Also one should select the journal that suits best with the paper. Manuscript should be prepared well. Review of the research is very important and some colleague or professor should review the paper. Submission should be followed by expecting the response. One should not be afraid of rejections.

Introduction

Publication is the essence of science something that scientists live everyday. In general, there is a general saying, "perform or perish" and it has been replaced in science by "publish or perish".

There is a genuine pressure that we feel on the people to publish. This tendency is increasing in India day by day. Majority of Indian medical institutions engage in medical research now and some of them are very productive. So learning how to publish is very important.

Getting Started

Often new students find it dauntingly hard to think of manuscripts. When randomly surveyed, Indian medical graduates trying to get hold of thesis topics will seem to be lost and have just more than a vague idea about research. That is because, they have no previous background and they all of sudden enter into unknown territory. Therefore, in the beginning guidance, clear directions and assistance is needed.

Select a Topic

Selecting a topic is difficult, because several thoughts come to mind. However, something that you have connected with right from beginning will help. For example, in pharmacology if you liked calcium channel blockers or arrhythmias in medicine or hernia in surgery or premenstrual tension in gynecology could be your broad thesis/manuscript papers. Often professors in India would like to start you with case reports or case series. If you get to write an original article early on in your career, you could be lucky.

Literature Search

Once you get an idea of the broad area; think of literature search. This will give you a better idea as to what others have done and what has been produced earlier. It may take lot of time (Fig. 37.1).

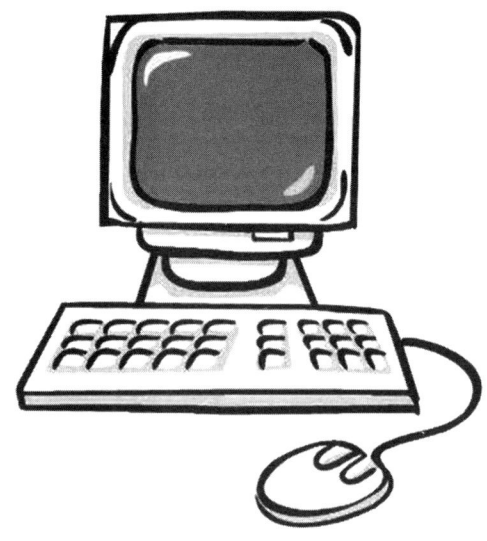

Fig. 37.1: Common search engines could be useful for gross search and defining the research question

Look into www.pubmed.com or www. google.com or www.googlescholar.com. Be aware if you are a China passed Indian medical graduate; then Google related applications do not work in general in China. They work nicely in India though. Look at full length articles if you interested in that topic seriously. Abstract contain only the concise information and are not enough!

Title/aim

If you writing a manuscript, select a short and informative title. It should be eye-catching one that gets the reader's attention! Short titles rather than long and explanatory are better. Keep the reader guessing rather than explaining everything in title itself.

Aim vs Objective

Aim is the ultimate outcome that one is seeking and the objective the way and means by which we shall achieve the same. Objectives can be many, but aim has to be one. Objectives can be primary and secondary. For the sake of simplicity; one should keep the objectives to minimum number. Sometimes when we become enthusiastic we may keep many of them but keeping them to 1–2 is better (Fig. 37.2).

Hypothesis

This is the backbone of your research and it should be thoughtfully crafted. Be prepared with null and alternative hypothesis. All major journals will look into this with *Google eyes*. They would want to know if you had formulated it correctly and if the results and discussion which has been presented actually match up to the same.

Research Question

This is an extension of your hypothesis and is it actually something that you are investigating and trying to find the answer of. A research question is the workable hypothesis that you are trying to find the answer of!

Material and Methods

This is the most valuable part of the paper which is read by serious readers. Indeed if they have been described nicely, then the results are going to be read as well (Fig. 37.3).

Else, most readers would stop here! Be descriptive, and express, "how can someone else do the same by reading the section you are describing". That means, it should be the "workable material and methods".

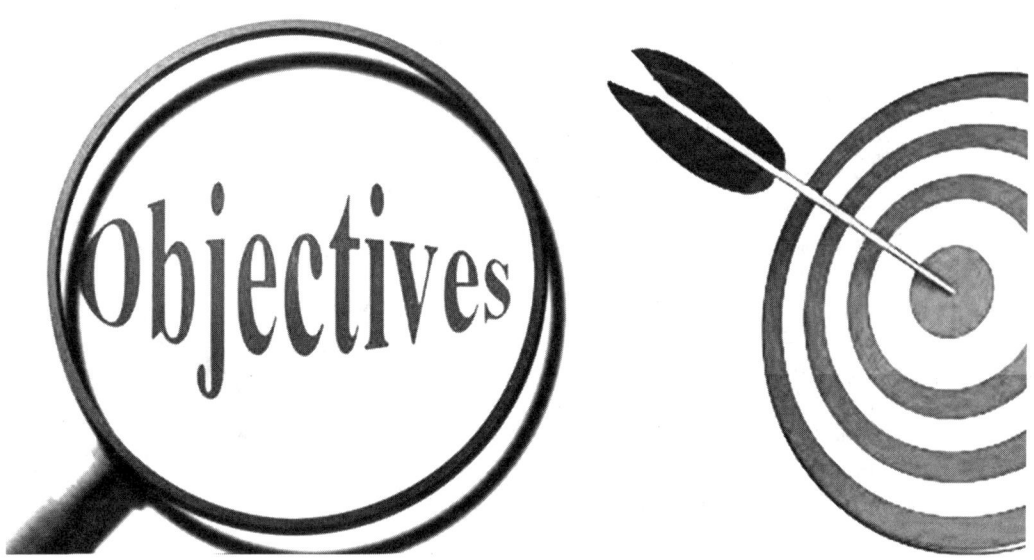

Fig. 37.2: Objective is the practical way in which the aim can be achieved

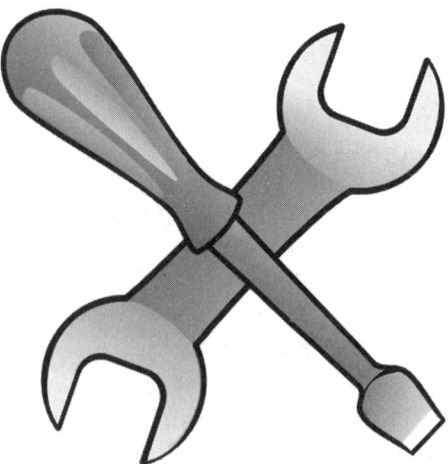

Fig. 37.3: Working on the manuscript is very important and it should be read many times before finalizing for publication. Every detail should be critically looked

Some journals want the same under following heads:

a. *Population*: What is the total number your studied? How did you select the population? How did you decide that this was a representative sample size? Was it a hospital based study or a community sample? (Fig. 37.4).

b. *Sample size*: Very important determinant of the study. It can be small or large. Was it a convenient sampling or was it something you selected based upon a formula. Was statistician consulted before the study began? How did you select alpha level (alpha) or beta level or power of the study?

c. *Consent*: Was informed consent taken and the process of taking the consent.

d. *Ethical approval*: Nowadays, it is important to take Ethical Committee approvals of the projects and one should have be explicit in this regard. In India, there is a clinical trial registry and it is important to have publication/s.

e. *Timelines*: If we were to submit a project, then the clear timelines will have to be submitted to funding agency.

f. *Budgets and audits*: Projects sponsored by pharmaceutical companies, will have to be submitted in detail and manpower, instruments, investigator fees, site charges, etc. will have to be explained in detail. Process of auditing will have to be clear.

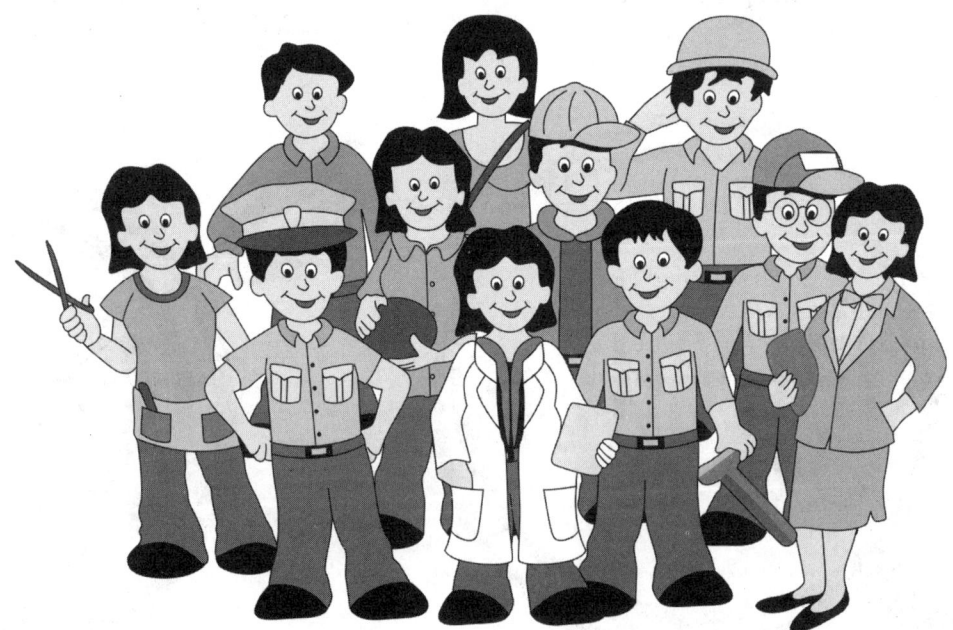

Fig. 37.4: Taking the right population for the study is the first step for achieving the goal

Discussion

This is most widely read part of paper where the researcher actually describes the same in detail. The results of the study are compared with the earlier. This will give the readers and idea as to how would your results be different from others.

Conclusion

This is an important part and should be kept short. One could describe the key findings and highlight the need for further research.

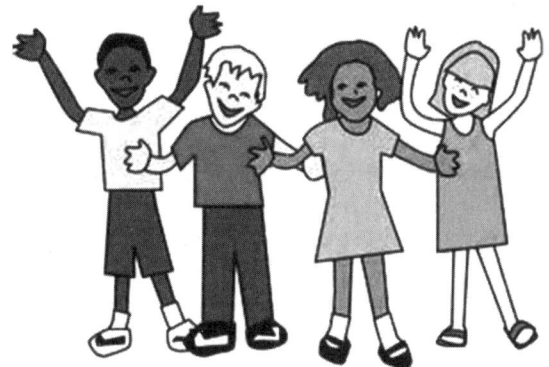

Fig. 37.5: Peer review can improve the quality of manuscript

Sending the Article to a Journal

Your guide will push you if you were doing MD/PhD/DM thesis and were trying to publish a paper to send your article in a good journal. Peer reviewed journals are good journals, especially the ones run by societies. Select one of those for you!

Most journals have online submissions nowadays and the websites are friendly. You just need to browse through the sites so that you can submit by being there and follow the instructions. There are options of going back and change something. So submission is an easy process. Make sure you have informed all your authors and your guides when you submitting a manuscript. All authors listen will get a submission email.

Peer Review

Most journals have this process where the journal article is sent for blind review. This is a simple process, where the experienced authors who have written manuscript earlier are made 'judges' and give blind comments on the manuscripts they have been sent. The comments sent by the reviewers are blind and detailed (Fig. 37.5).

They will have to be answered one by one. Please do not be intimated by extensive nature of comments and feel that your paper would be rejected. Even when comments are detailed and answered properly, the paper gets accepted! Eventually! However, one will have to persist and not to be disdained.

Answering Queries of Peer Reviewers

Peer review is a rigorous process and can be demotivating for the new scientists; for the seasoned scientists, it is a usual process that they sill through easily. One should answer the reviewers point by point and one has to be very objective about the same. One should preferably substantiate the same using some references. Even till last minute, reviewers and editors might want some corrections. Do not be discouraged by the same. Try to adhere to guidelines.

Getting Published

Normally, you are sent a proof of the paper before publishing. Even good journals can have error in manuscript; especially in titles, your names, addresses, affiliations, etc. so check the manuscript thoroughly before approving it for publication finally. Sometimes gross errors may be there and detected just at last minute!

Getting Linked with Google Scholar/ Research Gate

Several websites track the progress of researchers nowadays. One could make an account on one of these. These could calculate the *h-index, i-10 index* and number of citations in 5 years and also the impact points (research gate). In other words, your progress gets monitored automatically.

Deciding about the Author

An author is the person who has made substantial contribution to the paper. Generally, this is the person who has been involved at almost stages of the paper, i.e. inception, hypothesis, collecting information, executing study, collecting data and writing the report. Nowadays, it is not uncommon to see someone getting involved at a later stage. That means, someone could still come in at the editorial stage if the language of the paper needs major overhauling. Likewise, a statistician too can come at a later stages if the paper is unclear about the statistical methods used.

International committee of medical editors defines the author as following:

a. Involved from the conception and design of the manuscript.

b. Participated in interpretation of research findings.

c. Drafting of the article of revising the paper by providing the critical inputs needed for publication.

d. Final approval of the paper for publication.

e. Data collection alone, funding, general supervision does not alone qualify for the authorship.

Gifted Authorship

This is something that Indian authors are often confronted with. Whenever, a new manuscript is being prepared, there will always be some people around who would like to be the part of the same. One should however avoid the temptation of involving people in the same. In authors experience, the 'gifted authors' mostly do not value the manuscript and at some point or others will lead to problematic outcome.

Research Credits

Nowadays, it is common in Indian medical institutions to have publications as the basis of promotions. Slowly, it seems the "time bound" promotions will get replaced by a better system of 'credit based' promotions. Researchers get a score and based upon the same the researchers get promoted to medical and biomedical institutions.

Copyright

It is not uncommon to see at junior level specially to have infringement of copyright laws. Keep in mind, that if you copy someone else's work and make it look 'your own', its unethical. Be aware that this is a sub-standard practice and is never going to make you better researcher. Following should be kept in mind:

a. Cite the original author whenever, some material has been taken from his/her article.

b. Take due permission from author/ publisher or both when you are going to reproduce the work done by someone.

c. Before modifying some figure or flowchart, take permission from the authors.

d. Do not copy more than 6 lines, at a stretch and that too cite in the reference list or provide acknowledgment.

Plagiarism

This is an important issue in today's world with a large number of people interested in publications. There is a tremendous amount of race going on and hence, it is not uncommon to see people copying each other's work to get recognition. Plagiarism is simply copying the other's work to get recognition. It is therefore, important not to copy and write your own stuff! Plagiarism detecting software have now come and are able to identify if the manuscripts have been copied or not. Plagiarism is a major ethical offense!

Conflict of Interest

One has to declare if someone has some conflict of interest as to if someone accepted some favors from some company to write in their favors or modified the manuscript as per requirement. Though uncommon, but still one should declare this while writing a manuscript to a journal. It is generally expressed as:

Conflict of interest: None

This will save the scientist or medical doctor from participating in a manuscript whose results may be clouded.

Duplicate Publications

Someone may submit the paper to more than one journal and this is counted as a duplicate publication. One must not do this. In modern world, a journal will always ask if this paper has been published somewhere or is being considered somewhere for publication. This is another major ethical offense to have two papers which are identical!

Communicating to Press

Media in modern India is independent and proactive. They often reach out to the people in scientific world and ask them if anything new has happened. It is a common temptation to discuss things at length with people who are in press. However, if there is a finding that has been published in the peer review journal and has been well-documented should be communicated to the press. While such a communication is being done, care should be taken to do so in laymen language so that everyone can understand. Technical details should be avoided. Same goes true when a scientist or a medical doctor appears on TV or Radio shows.

Scientific Frauds

This is a rare event when a scientist or a medical doctor fabricates the results of the studies done by someone and then publishes the same under his or her name! This is a gross scientific misconduct. In some nations, for this behavior, even the name of the doctor can be struck from medical register records. In India, such issues are slowly getting addressed. Now, the medical editors active seek the articles that are original and check their originality. Moreover, most journals in Indian subcontinent will ask the contributors to submit a certificate that the work done is original and has not been copied. Likewise, it is also needed that an undertaking is given by the researchers that the work done has neither been not submitted nor been published anywhere.

Editorial Responsibilities

Editors have a major responsibility in ensuring the contents that they publish. It is prime concern of the biomedical editor that the material to be published has all the accurate contents. Additionally, they have to check for plagiarism as well. They have to ensure that the content that has been submitted to them is 'ethical' and has been scrutinized by the institutional ethical committees as well.

In India, in particular, nowadays, this is a growing challenge to be able to scrutinize manuscripts that come to the editors for publication. It is a full time job to ensure accuracy, check plagiarism and follow the individual ones to the logical conclusion.

Bibliography

1. Academic and professional writing. http://writing.wisc.edu/Handbook/Plan Research Paper.html (Downloaded on April 17th 2017).
2. How to write a research paper? http://www.wikihow.com/Write-a-Research-Paper (Downloaded on April 17th 2017).
3. Writing research papers for students. http://www.aresearchguide.com/1steps.html (Downloaded on April 17th 2017).

Evaluating the
Medical Literature

Learning objectives

One can start evaluating the research paper by examining the title. Like the question the paper deals with pertains well to the topic or issue that interests enough to spark thoughts and opinions? Also, is the question easily and fully researchable? The evaluation should be through and critical as to get the information one is seeking.

Introduction

Evaluating a scientific paper is a particular skill that one learns with the passage of time. However, the foundations are laid right in beginning.

At masters levels (MSc/MD) one should have develop a critical attitude towards evaluating the papers (Table 38.1).

The following general points should be kept in mind:

a. **Be skeptical:** Do not just blindly accept what has been published in a medical journal.

   In the beginning students are fond of quoting senior authors. On the one hand this is admirable as they have respect for someone who did something; on the other hand this trend of accepting something unscrupulously could be harmful also (Fig. 38.1).

b. **Raise questions:** How could the manuscript be written, read about material, methods, results and discussion part of the paper. A common error many student make is to just copy the abstract from the www.pubmed.com and then try to get the feel of whole paper (Fig. 38.2).

   Remember, while the trailer can give you an idea about the movie that is about

Table 38.1: Habits students must develop while evaluating research papers

- Read from critical angle
- Do not accept everything that has been published as the whole truth
- Remember, science is evolving

Unnecessary skepticism on everything could lead ignorance however

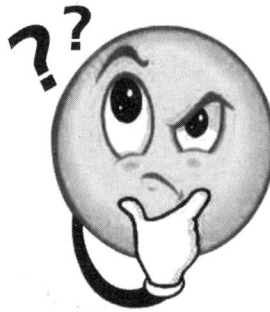

Fig. 38.1: One should always be raising questions rather than accepting things the way they are. Asking questions can always shed light on things not properly described

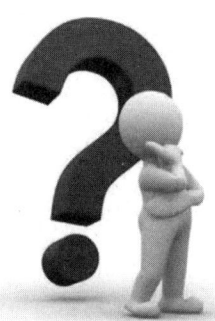

Fig. 38.2: Critical attitude is a must while evaluating medical literature

to come; but it is certainly not the complete movie. Therefore, do not just read abstract and be happy with this. Most good libraries in India will have a subscription of leading journals! Read them.

c. **Peer-review:** Though most of the journals in medicine and in biomedical sciences have this peer-review process and this is the norm; but still sometimes, some journals publish unscrupulous material that has not been properly scrutinized. This is particularly true of the "open access" journals. Remember, all of them are not bad; some of them may be! One good approach in authors experience is to "evaluate a paper, as if you have written it yourself" or "what different would you have done" in case you were the lead author or one of the co-author of the same.

When reading the paper, the following specific points should be kept in mind:

a. **Title:** An interesting title, or gripping headline is likely to get your attention. So catchy tittles are read more often that long detailed titles. Remember, "do not finish paper in the title itself". You have been given 1500–3000 words for a review of an original paper.

b. **Abstract:** It gives a clear idea about what is the aim, objective, results, discussion and conclusion the authors are trying to draw from the study samples. However, it should not be all as suggested previously. There is always more to a research paper than just the abstract. So if the paper interests you, certainly read the full-length. Do not just be satisfied with the abstract alone as full length may reveal surprising and interesting details.

c. **Material and methods:** For an interesting reader, it would always be the case that he/she will like to read material methods in details. There is a popular saying in medicine, i.e. A paper, whether it will sink of float, depends upon how good the material and methods has been written. Many papers contain methodological flaws hence have a lower retaining value compared to those which are descriptive.

d. **Repeat experiment if you can:** Sometimes, when you have been working on a particular topic and have read an interesting paper; results of this paper may quite different from your own. Do not panic! Try to reproduce the experiment using same methods described in the paper and see if your results also come same or they are different. This way, one can calculate the difference between two raters (inter-rater reliability). Obviously, two raters should not have a major difference. Likewise, difference in the readings of the same rater taken twice on two separate occasions is called intra-rater reliability. Goes without saying that both intra-rater and inter-rater reliability should be high.

e. **Statistics:** Most if not all of us, get put off by long lengthy statistical tests that authors use in their papers. Indeed this could be a deliberate ploy to give "cosmetic appeal" to the paper. Be aware! However, one need not to be a statistician to be able to analyze statistical tests. Elementary knowledge of statistics should help. One could see if authors have used any statistical method or not and if yes, has the selection been right or wrong! Naturally, wrong selection of test will not justify a right conclusion.

f. **Peer:** Reviewed journals: This is a journal that will submit its papers for outside review. Blind peer-review is considered to be the cornerstone of a sound scientific paper. Be aware of citing an unscrupulous journal that does not have a good reputation (calculated nowadays by impact factors, h-index and i-index). Impact factors are not calculated by scientists or medical doctors but by independent agencies like *Science Citation Index*. Some of the agencies like Journal Citation reports calculate the impact factors as following:

$$\text{Impact factor} = \frac{\text{Number of times article has been cited}}{\text{Total number of articles published during that period}}$$

Usually, the calculation is done for 2 years period.

In the peer-reviewed journals, all the essentials of peer-review as in blinding, conflict of interest, etc. are generally taken care of. It should be noted that merely circulation of a journal does not count. For example, nature has a circulation of 30,000 but an impact factor of 25 but the Journal of American Medical Association (JAMA) has a circulation of 3,70,000, which is more than 10 times of the nature but has an impact factor 3 times less! So technically, impact factor is not related to the quality of paper, but a good quality paper is likely to be cited more often.

g. **Reviews:** These are compilation of the published data and are not counted as "original articles". However, since the collect information from several sources; these have a great educational value and are perhaps the most commonly type of read educational material in scientific literature.

h. **Systematic reviews and meta-analysis:** Meta-analysis is a special form of systematic review in which the results are obtained by pooling the results of a large number of studies to get the defined outcome. Since a large number of studies are included to know the results of different investigations or interventions, sample size and power of the overall data is always more compared to the individual trial. Generally, pooling is done for a large number of similar studies. Care is taken not to include just the positive studies otherwise the results can be biased!

Bibliography

1. Check list for review reports. http://jan. ucc. nau.edu/pe/exs514web/How2Evalarticles. htm (Downloaded on April 17th 2017).

2. Evaluate your research question. https:// www.esc.edu/online-writing center/resources/ research/research-paper-steps/developing-questions/worksheet-evaluate-research-question/(Downloaded on April 17th 2017).

3. Evaluating published research. http://www. sciencedirect.com/science/article/pii/ S004873331500018 5 (Downloaded on April 17th 2017).

Effect Size

Effect size is medically relevant difference. In some researches, this is all that matters. To be able to interpret the effect size correctly, one should know the *p-value* and alpha level correctly. *P-Value* is the probability that the results were due to chance and *P-values* range from 0 to 1. The lower the *p-value*, the more likely it is that a difference occurred as a result of intervention if the research is a trial. **Alpha (α) level** is the error rate that one is willing to accept. Alpha is often set at 0.05 or 0.01. The alpha level is also known as the Type I error rate. An alpha of 0.05 means that one is willing to accept that there is a 5% chance that results are due to chance rather than to intervention if the research is a trial.

What is Effect Size?

Effect size is a statistical concept that measures the strength of the relationship between two variables on a numeric scale, i.e. it is the medically relevant difference between two variables.

For instance, if we have data on the height of men and women and we notice that, on average, men are taller than women, the difference between the height of men and the height of women is known as the *effect size*. The greater the effect size, the greater the height difference between men and women will be.

Statistic effect size helps us in determining if the difference between variables (e.g. height in this example) is real or if it is due to a change of factors. In hypothesis testing, several things are connected to effect size, e.g. power, sample size, and significance level, etc.

In meta-analysis, effect size is concerned with different studies and then combines all the studies into single analysis. In statistics analysis, the effect size is usually measured in three ways: (1) standardized mean difference, (2) odd ratio, (3) correlation coefficient.

Types of Effect Size

a. **Pearson r correlation:** Pearson r correlation has been developed by Karl Pearson, and it is most widely used in statistics. This parameter of effect size is denoted by r. The value of the effect size of Pearson r correlation varies between −1 to +1. According to Cohen, the effect size is low if the value of correlation coefficient r varies around 0.1, medium if r varies around 0.3, and large if r varies more than 0.5.

b. **Standardized means difference:** When a research study is based on the population mean and standard deviation, then the following method is used to know the effect size:

$$\theta = \frac{\mu_1 - \mu_2}{\sigma}$$

The effect size of the population can be known by dividing the two population mean differences by their standard deviation.

c. **Cohen's d effect size:** Cohen's d is known as the difference of two population means and it is divided by the standard deviation from the data. Mathematically Cohen's effect size is denoted by:

$$d = \frac{\bar{x}_1 - \bar{x}_2}{s}$$

Where s can be calculated using this formula:

$$s = \sqrt{\frac{(n_1 - 1)s_1^2 + (n_2 - 1)s_2^2}{n_1 + n_2}}$$

d. **Glass's Δ method of effect size:** This method is similar to the Cohen's method, but in this method standard deviation is used for the second group. Mathematically this formula can be written as:

$$\Delta = \frac{\overline{x}_1 - \overline{x}_2}{s_2}$$

e. **Hedges' g method of effect size:** This method is the modified method of Cohen's d method. Hedges' g method of effect size can be written mathematically as follows:

$$g = \frac{\overline{x}_1 - \overline{x}_2}{s*}$$

Where standard deviation can be calculated using this formula:

$$\text{Std. Deviation} = \sqrt{\frac{s_1^2(n_1 - 1) + s_2^2(n_2 - 1)}{n_1 + n_1 - 2}}$$

Odd ratio: The odds ratio is the odds of success in the treatment group relative to the odds of success in the control group. This method is used in cases when data is binary.

The odds-ratio and risk-ratio effect sizes (OR and RR) are designed for contrasting two groups on a binary/dichotomous dependent variable. It can be computed from 2 by 2 frequency tables or from outcome event proportions for each group. With the marginal distributions, it can be comptued from a chi-square and a phi coefficient.

Interpreting Effect Size

Effect sizes are usually reported using the label size difference or 'd'. It is given in the form of decimal value like 0.1, 0.2, 0.3, etc. One of the most common ways of interpreting effect sizes is based on the work of a Cohen who defined effect size quantitatively. He said 0.2 and below = small effect size; 0.5 = medium effect size; 0.8 and above = large effect size.

Cohen's suggestions are generally accepted and are a good basis for interpreting the results of trials and in reading systematic reviews and meta-analyses.

Effect Size and Statistical Significance

Statistical significance, tells us if an intervention had an effect that was unlikely to have happened by chance. While it is important to know this, it is not as useful for comparing effect sizes of multiple studies, as we do in systematic reviews. This is because statistical significance does not take into account sample size. If two studies are identical except that one has a larger sample size, we would usually consider the study with the larger sample size to be more reliable. Statistical significance does not give more weight to a study with more participants, i.e. all studies are treated equally.

Effect sizes, on the other hand, are 'weighted' according to the number of participants in a study. For instance, a study with 10 participants might have had a big effect size (such as 0.8); while another study of the same intervention may have had 1000 participants but a small effect size (such as 0.2). If all other things are equal (e.g. both studies had a low risk of bias), then both studies may have shown that the intervention had a statistically significant effect, but the overall effect size would be small, because the larger of the two studies would be given more 'weight'.

A Forest Plot

A forest plot is a graphical representation of a meta-analysis. It is usually accompanied by a table listing references (author and date) of the studies included in the meta-analysis. In the example here, there were three studies included in the meta-analysis: Dhikav 2011, Dhikav and Anand 2010 and Dhikav 2013. The table also lists the mean scores and standard deviations of these scores from each of the included studies; and it lists the number of participants in each study.

The forest plot is the graph on the right-hand side. It has one line representing each study in the meta-analysis, plotted according to the Standardised Mean Difference (SMD).

This is the difference between the average score of participants in the intervention group, and the average score of participants in the control group.

Interpreting the forest plot involves two steps:

a. Determine effect size
b. Level of difference or heterogeneity among different trials in meta-analysis.

a. *Effect Size*

One would have to determine where does the black diamond sit between the set effect size. For example, if it sits half way between 0 and −1, then effect size is 0.5. According to a common interpretation of effect sizes, this would suggest that the intervention being tested in these three studies had a small to medium effect size—in other words, 'it worked' and had a moderate effect. This depends upon if this effect size goes towards (favors intervention).

In addition to the effect size, it is also important to consider the level of heterogeneity in a meta-analysis.

b. *Heterogeneity*

Systematic reviews and meta-analyses aim to capture the overall effects of an intervention or treatment when it has been tested in multiple trials. Ideally, if multiple trials are testing the same intervention, the effects of the

intervention should be consistent across all of the studies. Unfortunately, this is rarely the case, because many things can affect the results of a trial, such as researcher bias, problems with data collection, or any number of other things.

Systematic review and meta-analysis are designed to ask a common question, i.e. if studies are all testing the same intervention, why do not they get the same results? Are the differences caused by chance, or is there something else involved? If it is the former, then we can have confidence in the results of the meta-analysis. If the differences are not the result of chance, then we need to be cautious in interpreting the results of the meta-analysis.

Fortunately, it is easy to tell if heterogeneity is due to chance (or not) by interpreting the I^2 **statistic**. An I^2 statistic of more than 50% is considered high.

Bibliography

1. Power Analysis, Statistical Significance, and Effect Size. http://meera.snre.umich.edu/power-analysis-statistical-significance-effect-size (Accessed online on 3rd March 2017).
2. Practical Meta-Analysis Effect Size Calculator. https://www.campbellcollaboration.org/escalc/html/EffectSizeCalculator-Home.php (Accessed online on 3rd March 2017).
3. Statistics solutions. http://www.statisticssolutions.com/statistical-analyses-effect-size/ (Accessed online on 3rd March 2017).

Survival Analysis

Learning objectives

Survival analysis is set of methods for data analysis where the outcome variable is the time until the occurrence of an event. The event can be birth, death, disease, marriage, divorce, etc. The outcome variable is the time until an event occurs. Time could be measured in years, months, weeks, or days, etc. the survival analysis starts from day (0) the follow-up till event. The event could be death, disease, relapse, recovery, etc. Time is taken as the survival time and it indicates the time that an individual has survived over some follow-up period. The event of interest usually is death, disease or any other negative individual experience.

Why do Survival Analysis?

Survival analysis helps the researcher assess if, any why, certain individuals are exposed to a higher risk of experiencing an event of interest, such as death, machine failure, drug relapse, etc. This is also referred to as event history analysis. Survival analysis consists of a wide variety of techniques that help the researcher analyze time-to-event models. Survival analysis can be used to study many things and is extremely helpful in studying the cause of births and deaths. It can also be used by the researcher in order to understand the cause(s) of marriages and divorces, and even the cause of wars and revolutions.

WHAT IS SURVIVAL ANALYSIS?

Survival analysis is referred to statistical methods for analyzing survival data. Survival data could be derived from laboratory studies of animals or from clinical and epidemiologic studies, etc. Survival data could relate to outcomes for studying acute or chronic diseases.

Survival Time

Survival time refers to a variable which measures the time from a particular starting time (e.g. time initiated the treatment) to a particular endpoint of interest (e.g. attaining certain functional abilities). It is important to note that for some subjects in the study a complete survival time may not be available due to censoring. Some patients may still be alive or in remission at the end of the study period. The exact survival times of some subjects are unknown. These are called *censored observation* or *censored times* and can also occur when individuals are lost to follow-up after a period of study.

Censoring

Censoring means a person does not experience the event before the study ends. It means a person is lost to follow-up during the study. A person withdraws from the study because of death (if death is not the event of interest) or some other reason.

Uses of Survival Analysis

a. Clinical trials (e.g. recovery time after heart surgery)
b. Longitudinal or cohort studies (e.g. time to observing the event of interest)
c. Life insurance (e.g. time to file a claim)
d. Quality control and reliability in manufacturing (e.g. the amount of force needed to damage a part such that it is not useable).

Survival Function

Let T denote the survival time so $S(t) = P$ (surviving longer than time t)

$$= P(T > t)$$

The function S(t) is also known as the cumulative survival function. S(t) = number of patients surviving longer than t = total number of patients in the study.

Kaplan-Meier Plot

Kaplan-Meier estimate is one of the best options to be used to measure the fraction of subjects living for a certain amount of time after treatment. In clinical trials the effect of an intervention is assessed by measuring the number of subjects survived or saved after that intervention over a period of time. The time starting from a defined point to the occurrence of a given event for example, death is called survival time and the analysis of group data as survival analysis. This can be affected by subjects under study that are uncooperative and refused to be remained in the study or when some of the subjects may not experience the event or death before the end of the study, although they would have experienced or died if observation continued, or we lose touch with them midway in the study.

The Kaplan-Meier estimate is the simplest way of computing the survival overtime in spite of all these difficulties associated with subjects or situations. The survival curve can be created assuming various situations. It involves computing of probabilities of occurrence of event at a certain point of time and multiplying these successive probabilities by any earlier computed probabilities to get the final estimate. This can be calculated for two groups of subjects and also their statistical difference in the survivals. The following questions can be answered by this: like what proportion of a given population will survive past a set date?

Of the population that survived, what is the rate they will die/fail? Or do certain factors (e.g. age and gender) effect the probability of survival? Survival analysis is represented in Fig. 40.1.

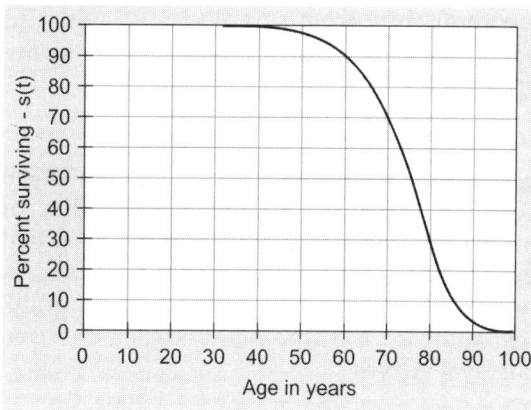

Fig. 40.1: Representative curve for all cause mortality

Steps for Kaplan-Meier Analysis

The first step in survival analysis is for the researcher to establish what event is to be analyzed. For example, suppose in a study of marital histories, four types of states are obtained: 'never married,' 'married,' 'divorced,' and 'widowed.' The term 'event' is a transition from one state to another. In this example, the event can be referred to as 'married,' which is a transition from the origin of 'never married' to the final state of 'married.' The next step is to ensure that the data consists of a longitudinal record of when the event has occurred for individuals or group of individuals. Using the example above, this may include ages and marriage dates, as well as other explanatory variables (e.g. gender, income, etc.).

The dependent variable can be survival time or transition rate, and analyses can be conducted to describe the varying proportions of surviving cases at different times or to assess the relationship between survival time and a set of covariates/predictors.

The most common event analyzed in survival analysis is death. Other common events are unemployment, graduation from school, machine failure, etc. The survival time data in survival analysis has two important special characteristics. The survival time data in survival analysis is not negative and is usually positively skewed.

The survival time, which is the object of study in survival analysis, should be differentiated from the calendar time. The survival time in survival analysis should always be measured related to some appropriate time origin.

Longrank Test

SPSS, SAS, S-plus and many other statistical software packages have the capability of analyzing survival data. Logrank Test can be used to compare two survival curves. A *p-value* of less than 0.05 based on the logrank test indicate a difference between the two survival curves.

Hazard Function

The hazard function *h(t)* of survival time *T* gives the *conditional failure rate*. The hazard function is also known as the *instantaneous failure rate, force of mortality,* and *age-specific failure rate. It gives the risk of failure per unit time during the aging process.*

Multivariate analysis: Cox's Proportional Hazards Model (CPHM) is a technique for investigating the relationship between survival time and independent variables. A proportional hazard model possesses the property that different individuals have hazard functions that are proportional to one another.

Bibliography

1. http://stats.idre.ucla.edu/stata/dae/multivariate-regression-analysis/(Accessed online on dated 2nd May 2017).

2. http://www.camo.com/multivariate_analysis. html (Accessed online on dated 2nd May 2017).

3. Introduction to multivariate analysis. https://www.jmp.com/support/help/13-1/Introduction_to_Multivariate_Analysis.shtml (Accessed online on dated 2nd May 2017).

Uncontrolled Clinical Trials

Learning objectives

An open clinical trial or an uncontrolled is a clinical trial without a control group, as opposed to a controlled clinical trial which has a comparison group. It can also be a non-blinded clinical trial, as opposed to a single-blind or double-blind clinical trial. Early clinical studies of new and untried therapies could be done using uncontrolled clinical trials. Uncontrolled clinical trials represent early phase studies where the standard is relatively ineffective. This design is particularly good for investigations which cannot be done within the current climate of controversy (no "clinical equipoise"). Few clinical researchers label uncontrolled clinical trial, as a clinical trial, a before–after design, a screening design, or an intervention study.

Introduction

Many clinical trials are done without a control groups and are known as uncontrolled trials. Since, there is a lack of comparison group, therefore, they convey less information. In early stages of clinical research, they may play an important role. They however could be succeeded by the large scale clinical trials to confirm the same.

Essentially, an uncontrolled study is a study in which all the participants are given a treatment and simply followed for a period of time to see if they improve, with no comparison against another group (control group) that is either taking another treatment or no treatment at all. This is a simplistic alternative to the more complicated randomized clinical trials.

It has been discussed earlier that clinical trials form the basis of evidence-based medicine. The primary aim of clinical trials is to provide an unbiased estimate of the evaluation of two drug therapies or intervention.

Naturally, our aim is to make sure that the two group comparison is free from any kind of bias. This may however not always be possible. One effective way of doing this is to achieve randomization. Other could be matching. The latter could ensure that the two are evenly matched in their baseline characteristics.

At times, however, our aim is just to show the efficacy of a group and we do not want to show superiority of one group over the other. Therefore, we may not need a control group there. *Uncontrolled trials* could be done in such cases. These trials may be non-randomized as a comparison group is not utilized. So overall, all patients in uncontrolled trials are given same form of treatment as the patients did not have a comparison group.

Place of Uncontrolled Trials in Therapeutics

A controlled variable remains constant and does not change throughout an experiment, while the term "uncontrolled" applies to studies where one cannot be certain that their test subjects are receiving the treatment in question or not. Evidence-gathered during uncontrolled studies can thus be inconclusive and controlled trials are hence needed.

Why Perform an Uncontrolled Trial?

An open label trial has no control group as opposed to the controlled trial which has. It can be a non-blind trial where an investigator knows everything about the same.

It goes without saying that clinical trials that are double blind, randomized and placebo control could be the best form of treatment given. Therefore, it is important that wherever possible, these are the preferred form of treatments. However, in certain situations, uncontrolled trials may be more appropriate:

a. Demonstrate pharmacokinetic activity of a drug in Phase I trial.
b. Generate hypothesis for further clinical research.

In phase I trial, a control group or comparison group is not needed. As the pharmacokinetic details of the drug have not been established. Many pharmaceutical companies when introducing new combinations; go for pharmacokinetic details of the drugs in healthy volunteers. We wish to know:

a. Pharmacokinetic details like half-life, route of drug elimination, any metabolite, etc. in human beings for the first time.
b. Know maximal tolerated dose of the drug.

Authors conducted a phase II trial of yoga as a treatment modality in improving male sexual functions. This trial was done using International Index of Erectile Functions (IIEF), which is a standard tool to evaluate the drugs in erectile dysfunction. Authors did a before and after study and same group served as their own control. However, it did not have a control. Since, this was a first time trial of yoga; reviewers and editors felt that, the term, "uncontrolled" should be introduced in the title to give clear impression that this trial is uncontrolled.

After this study has been done, several similar studies have been done as well. So this study being the seminal study served to generate the hypothesis that such trials could be used to further the hypothesis or confirm the same.

If it is unethical to include "sham group"; then uncontrolled trials are the only trials possible. Before and after treatment evaluation can however be done. Likewise, in oncology, toxic treatments are tried. Therefore, demonstrating efficacy may be taken as an evidence without comparing (Sacca L, 2010).

Disadvantage: Main limitation of uncontrolled trials is that they need to be confirmed in large studies (Table 41.1).

Table 41.1: Strengths of uncontrolled trials

Strengths	Weakness
Generate hypothesis	Investigator bias may occur as investigators may believe in their own treatments
Provide ground for large scale treatment	Interpretation could be difficult and may not be a informative as the controlled trials
If it is unethical to include a control group, then one can go ahead	Concurrent control group provides best chance of interpreting the results as immediate comparison is available

Conclusions

Uncontrolled trials have an important role in clinical research and provide a ground for evaluating new and untested treatments. They often serve to generate sufficient evidence for further exploration of trials. If it is unethical to include a control group, e.g. in surgical trials; uncontrolled trails with before and after evaluation could be the best method evaluation.

Bibliography

1. Controlled and uncontrolled studies. https://faculty.unlv.edu/beisecker/Courses/Phi-102/Controlled_Studies.htm (Downloaded on April 17th 2017).
2. Dhikav V, Karmarkar G, Verma M, Gupta R, Gupta S, Mittal D, Anand K. Yoga in male sexual functioning: a noncomparative pilot study. J Sex Med. 2010 Oct; 7(10):3460–3466.
3. Saccà L. The uncontrolled clinical trial: scientific, ethical, and practical reasons for being. Intern Emerg Med. 2010 Jun;5(3):201–4. doi: 10.1007/s11739–010-0355-z.

Research Integrity

Learning objectives

This is a new area of concern in medical research. Public concerns over research misconduct initially arose in the early 1980's. At the time, research institutions sometimes ignored or covered up potential misconduct problems rather than investigate them. In India, it has been dealt by issuing light warnings only. By the year 2000 polices started coming about research misconduct in industrialized nations. The issue is getting attention in India too.

Introduction

Common principals of research integrity include honesty in all aspects of research, accountability in the conduct of research and professional courtesy and fairness in working with others. Good stewardship of research on behalf of others is important.

The Department of Health and Human Services, USA defines research misconduct as fabrication, falsification, or plagiarism in proposing, performing, or reviewing research results.

Fabrication is, simply stated, making up results and recording or reporting them.

Falsification on the other hand is manipulation of research materials, equipment, or processes, or changing or omitting results such that the research is not accurately represented in the record.

Plagiarism (as detailed elsewhere also) is the copying of another's ideas, processes, results, or words without giving proper credit.

Research misconduct represents a significant departure from accepted practices. Has been committed intentionally, or knowingly, or recklessly; and can be proven by a preponderance of evidence. However, what is not misconduct is the honest, unintentional error.

Frequency of Research Misconduct
(Table 42.1)

Research misconduct is not common; however, some examples keep coming. How often does scientific misconduct occur is an important question? There seems to be no consensus on the answer. To raise ethical standards, program to investigate the prevalence of fraud, data fabrication, plagiarism, and other questionable practices in science, grants have now been approved.

Table 42.1: Common lapses in research integrity
- Failure to report all data
- Fabrication of data number
- Falsification of data on study report forms
- Non reporting of adverse drug reactions

In some countries like US, there seems to be a recent increase in frequency in last decade or so. Hence, a need was felt to investigate its actual frequency.

Types of Research Misconduct

Since, this is a new form of behavior, more is being learnt. However, lot of types have been investigated so far. Given below is a general introduction:

a. **Data cooking:** This is falsifying or 'cooking' research data and is not uncommon. This means, without doing actual experiments, results are made.

b. **Not following protocol:** Ignoring major aspects of human-subject requirements in medical research.

c. **Non disclosure:** Not properly disclosing involvement in firms whose products are based on one's own research. This seems to be a growing trend nowadays.

d. **Illicit relations:** Relationships with students, research subjects or clients that may be interpreted as questionable are not uncommon.

e. **Stealing ideas:** Using another's ideas without obtaining permission or giving due credit (plagiarism). Unauthorized use of confidential information in connection with one's own research also constitutes stealing.

f. **Canceling:** Failing to present data that contradict one's own/previous research and circumventing certain minor aspects of human-subject requirements could be questionable.

Addressing Research Misconduct in India

Research integrity officer receives complaint in many countries. In India, it is usually guide/dean/director do so. Complainant is then sent to the research committee and the candidate is interviewed by the inquiry committee. Candidate is notified in writing of the allegation and pertinent data records are examined. Any individuals pertinent to the investigation could also be interviewed by the committee. Research committee submits findings and recommendations to the guide/dean/director, who decides about the quantum of punishment.

If research misconduct has been found, the deciding authority determines what administrative actions are appropriate and reports to the vice chancellor of the university.

Conclusions

The aim of research training is the responsible conduct of research and to promote a general awareness of professional norms in scientific research. Also, research training aims to encourage a life-long attention to the ethical principles from which they are derived. Hence, research professionals are duty bound to follow research ethics.

Bibliography

1. Research Integrity https://www.research.vt.edu/reports/Research_Misconduct. (Accessed online on July 6th 2017).
2. Research integrity. http://graduateschool.uncc.edu/sites/graduateschool.uncc.edu/files/media/CRS/RCR-2015.pdf (Accessed online on July 6th 2017).
3. Research Integrity-John Hopkins University. www.hopkinsmedicine.org/research/.../Research_Integrity/.../DeansRILecture7_03282 (Accessed online on July 6th 2017).

Appendix 1
Commonly Used Terms in Medical Research

ABSOLUTE VALUE

This the value of the number, regardless of the sign. It is denoted by a pair of " | " signs. It is dependent upon modulus. For example, the modulus of –2.5 is $|-2.5| = 2.5$.

Alternative Hypothesis

When we conduct clinical trials, we start with a negative assumption that there is no difference [H_0] between the (test) and (control). However, it may turn out to be false, then we have to reject the null hypothesis.

Null and alternative hypothesis

$$- H_0 = Mu_1 = Mu_2$$
$$- H_1 = Mu_1 \neq Mu_2$$

Average

This is a commonly used term for the middle value. It is usually interpreted as the mean. However, it may also infer median. One should be clear about the use of loose terms in statistics.

Assumptions (Statistical)

Certain assumptions are kept in statistics and followed through. In statistics, the aim to estimate population parameters using the sample parameters and these will hold true only when sample parameters and assumptions have been followed correctly. Generally, we assume that the data will follow a normal distribution. This however, will be applicable only when explicitly stated and sample size is sufficiently large.

Bar Chart

This type of chart shows frequencies of a variable that is categorical or discrete. The height of bars are proportional to the frequencies or percentages. This is a very basic type of expression used in clinical medicine to show a variety of data. In between the bars, there is a space. Width has to be equal.

Binomial Distribution

If the data set that we are analyzing has only two categories, e.g. hot or cold or tall and short, then this type of data shows binomial distribution. This is used to model data from categorical variables when there are just two data set. This is used for mutually exclusive events. That means, on a given cloudy day, bright sunshine and high humid temperature is not expected. So two events are mutually exclusive.

Formula of calculating probability is:

$$p(y) = \frac{x}{y} \ p^y \left(1 - p\right)^{n-y}$$

n = Number is sample
$y = 0,1, ..., n$
p = Probability of y
$p(y)$ = Probability distribution of y

Standard error and confidence interval of the estimate of probability can be given.

Boxplot ("Box and Whisker" Plot)

Tukey introduced this more than 40 years back and is a graphical representation of numerical data based upon 5 number summary. This diagram has a scale in one direction only.

It consists of a rectangular box extending from the lower quartile to upper quartile. A median is shown dividing the box. Whisker are then drawn extending from the box from greatest and least value. Multiple box plots lying side by side can be used for comparison of multiple samples.

Whiskers may have a length not exceeding 1.5 times of the inter-quartile range. Any value that extends beyond the whiskers are shown as outliers. Any value beyond 3 times of inter-quartile range will be interpreted as extreme outlier.

Categorical Variable

Any variable that does not have numerical values and is being presented just by categories only. This could be: males, females, fat, thin, etc. probability distribution for statistical analysis used could be binomial distribution.

CENTRAL LIMIT THEOREM

This is the backbone of whole of statistics. We all know that we calculate a fraction of the parameters and wish to extend this result to the population. There has to be a statistical backing for being able to do so. There is! And it is called central limit theorem. This assumes that if you were to calculate the sample statistics (x) and compare this from population mean (μ); there is an important truth here, i.e. if sample size is sufficiently large, then sample and population means could be equal.

Confidence Interval

This is an interval containing the variable of interest. This interval gives us the range in which the variable of interest is most likely to lie.

Continuous Variable

This is always a numerical value that make take any value within interval. This will give rise to continuous data, which is the highest form of data and can be subjected to inferential statistical tests easily. Height, weight and temperature are continuous variables.

In descriptive statistics, this may not be very important as same summary measures like mean, median, mode and standard deviation can be used.

This may however be important for inferential statistics as the tests that we use for analysis are based upon different assumptions and are more appropriate for continuous variables.

Cumulative Frequency Graph

For a given numerical variable, frequency corresponding to a number (x) is total number of observations that are less or equal to x. Y-axis can show frequency, or proportion or the percentage like bar chart. With the percentage, the graph shows any percentile to be read from the graph.

Decile

Introduced by Galton over 100 years back; deciles are used to divide a numerical variable into 10 parts like quartile divides it into 4 and percentile into 100 parts. Cumulative frequency curve helps us reading the value of deciles.

Descriptive Statistics

This is a branch of statistics dealing with exploration of data and use summary measures such as means, quartiles, etc. this also involves use of graphs, e.g. boxplot for data depiction. This type of data can be used to describe the data; generalization about larger population needs inferential statistics.

Discrete Variable

This is an example of data set that can be counted. For example, number of doctors doing duties in emergencies, number of medical students taking interest in medical research and gynecologists writing research papers annually, etc.

Dispersion

This is same as variability. Measures, such as standard deviations tell about the data spread and its distance from the mean.

Dot Plot

This is an alternative to boxplot where each of the value is represented by a dot. It is used for fewer data values. Dots may be jittered so that values may be visible. They may also be stacked to produce histogram. This is less commonly used. In a simple dot plot the dots may overlap. In some cases they may coincide completely, so obscuring some of the points. A solution is to randomly move the dots perpendicularly from the axis, to separate them from one another. This is called jittering. It results in a jittered dot plot.

Estimation

Process by which a sample data can be used to estimate the value of a unknown variable in the population.

These can be expressed as a single value called a point estimate. It is usual to give precision of estimate and is called standard error. Confidence interval with estimate will make estimation even more objective by indicating how much confident the researcher is about the estimate given.

Estimator

It is a quantity calculated from sample data and is used to give information about the unknown quantity which is usually a parameter in population.

Estimators are sometimes differentiated from true or population values. Like for example, x is sample mean and mu is population mean.

Five-number Summary

In a boxplot, sometimes values are shown as least value, lower and upper quartile, median and greatest value.

Summaries Minimum Lower

Quartile
Median upper
Quartile
Maximum

Factor

This is a common word for categorical variables. See factor analysis also.

Fisher

Fisher **(1890–1962)** was an English statistician; arguably the most influential statistician of the twentieth century. He was educated at Harrow and at Cambridge University, where he studied mathematics.

He was originally interested in genetics but later turned to statistics. However, he persued both of these interests for rest of his life. In his first paper he describe maximum likelihood. Then later he described t-distribution and correlation coefficient. Later following First World War, he worked upon F distribution and ANOVA. In one conference in India in 1958, he said workers in research should visit statistician before starting their work and not after that, "else is going to be a postmortem of data".

Frequencies

It is the number of times that the particular values are obtained in given variable.

The frequency is the number of times that particular values are obtained in a variable.

Doctors in neurology department	Frequency of emergency calls/weekly
Doctor A	3
Doctor B	5
Doctor C	3

GALTON (SIR FRANCIS 1822–1911)

Galton was an explorer and statistician having special interest in meterology.

Greek Letters

In statistics, greek letters are used for the parameters of the population and for a few other things.

The table below gives the pronunciation of those that are most used.

Greek letter used as symbols in statistics
Alpha level (α),
Intercept in regression line $y = \alpha + \beta x$
Beta level (β),
Slope in regression line $y = \alpha + \beta x$

Kai χ_2 test is a much (over) used significance test (χ)

[*Mu*] mean of the population (μ)

Pai the value is = 3.14 (π)

Also sometimes used for the population proportion

Theta used for the population proportion (θ)

Rho Correlation coefficient of the population (ρ)

Sigma Standard deviation of the population (σ)

Variance of the population (σ^2)

Sigma Shorthand for "The sum of" (Σ)

HYPOTHESIS TEST

This is the most important part of inferential statistics. One has to formulate both null (H_0) and alternative hypothesis (H_1) before proceeding with hypothesis testing.

If there is no difference then, $H_0 = H_1$, accept null hypothesis. If $H_0 \neq H_1$ then reject null and accept alternative hypothesis.

Inference

Analysis of data in and to be able to apply this data to population is one of the foremost aim. Many studies are just descriptive and inference is the process of deducing properties of distribution by data analysis. Some would say, it is the process of making generalizations about population using some sample data.

Inter-quartile Range

Interquartile range, which is an important tool for knowing data distribution was first used by Galton in 1882. Interquartile range is the difference between the upper and lower quartiles. If the lower and upper quartiles are denoted by Q1 and Q3, respectively, the interquartile range is (Q3–Q1).

Line Graph

This is a type of line diagram mad upon a scatter plot where individual points are connected by a line. Line will tell about the sequence in time, space or some other quantity. A line graph is a scatter plot where individual points are connected by a line.

Levels

Number of categories in a categorical variable. For example, there may be three categories in the categorical variable [type of services provided by a hospital]: Good, better, best.

Maximum

Highest value of a numerical variable. For example, in a score of a test medical students, 67, 78, 89, 90, 56, 77, 92 is the score. In this series, 92 is the highest value.

Mean

This is the most common measure of middle value. It is commonly called "average". However, "mean" is more appropriate as the term average may sometimes also be used for median. This is common denoted by symbol x when we deal with sample mean.

To calculate the mean, sum μ all the individual data values, and divide by their total number. For example, with the 7 values 12, 15, 11, 18, 13, 14, 18, the mean is:

$(12x = +15 + 11 + 18 + 13 + 14 + 18)/7$
$= 101/7 = 14.4$

The mean is given by the formula:
$$x = \Sigma x/n$$
where, Σ is short for "the sum of", "x" signifies that each value is taken in turn, and n is the number of observations.

Mean Deviation

This is a common measure of spread of data. Often it is stated as mean of the distance that each value has from the mean. It is given by the formula:

Mean deviation = $\Sigma x - x/(n-1)$

The mean deviation is an average (mean) difference from the mean. The value it gives is similar, but slightly smaller than the standard deviation. Although it is simpler than the standard deviation it is used less commonly. The reason is because the standard deviation, σ, is used in inference, because the population standard deviation, σ, is one of the parameters of the normal distribution.

For example, there are 9 residents in the Department of Neurology and their mean height is 170 centimeters. Now, if two more visiting doctors from a different institute come to join positing for a few days; and their individual heights are 160 and 165 centimeters. Then mean deviation from the mean of heights of doctors will be:

Mean height of doctors = 170 cm	Height of visiting doctor = 160, 160 cm
Mean deviation of doctor-1	170–160 = 10 cm
Mean deviation of doctor-2	170–165 = 5 cm

That means, mean deviation tells us about the distance of individual values from the mean. Since standard deviation is used in inferential statistics; therefore is less popular.

Median

Commonly interpreted as the "middle value" of a data that has been arranged in ascending or descending order. If the data has an even number then, middle two values are summed up and divided into two.

For example, with the same 7 values shown for the mean and maximum above the sorted data are as follows: 10, 20, 30, 45, 55, 39, 70. The median is therefore the 4th value in the sorted list, i.e. 45.

Minimum

The maximum is the lowest value in a numerical variable. In the variable with the values 10, 20, 30, 45, 55, 39, 70. Then 10 is the minimum value.

Mixed Variable

In some studies some variables are categorical and some are numerical.

In a study of patients attending dementia clinic, following was the data:

Patient type	Mini-mental state score (MMSE)	Serum cortisol
Mild dementia	22	10 mcg/dl
Moderate dementia	23	20 mcg/dl
Severe dementia	7	35 mcg/dl

Model (Statistical)

"Model" word is used in many ways. In statistics, this is usually a mathematical equation is used to "fit" the data best.

For example, there are many predictors of stroke, e.g. hypertension, hypercholesterolemia, obesity and diabetes. Now presence of one or more will increase the risk. Now, how do we know, as to what extent will the risk increase? A risk score model can be developed depending upon presence of risk factors.

Normal Distribution

This type of distribution is used for continuous variables. Properties of normal distribution are as follows:

a. The normal distribution is used to model some continuous variables. It is a symmetrical bell-shaped curve that is completely determined by two parameters. They are the population mean (μ), and the standard deviation (σ).

b. Most values (66%) are distributed around mean ± standard deviation.

c. This follows central limit theorem and predicts that the probability of finding a variable will fall between two numbers.

d. Larger the sample size, possibility that normal distribution exists is high.

In a normal distribution

$$y = \frac{1}{\sqrt{2\pi}} e^{-(x-\mu)^2}/2\sigma$$

μ = Mean
σ = Standard deviation
$\pi \approx 3.14159$
$e \approx 2.71828$

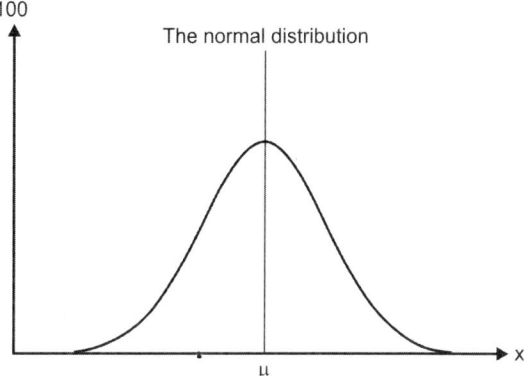

The normal distribution

Null Hypothesis

This is called the hypothesis of no difference. This assumes that there is no differences between cases and controls. Later on, as experiment progresses there may actually be a difference; then, we have to reject null hypothesis and accept the alternative hypothesis.

n-1

We use sample variance and standard deviation to calculate population variance and standard deviation. If you use *n*, and not *n-1*, population variance gets underestimated. *n-1* makes it unbiased estimator, which is desirable in inferential statistics.

Numerical Variable

This deals with numbers, like 15 medical students, 100 patients 200 blood samples, etc. Categorical variables on the other hand deals with categories like males and females, etc.

Ordinal Variable

This is a categorical type of data used in descriptive studies and deals with categories, e.g. strongly agree, disagree, etc. similarly, if we grade a swelling as small, medium and large that will also be an ordinal variable.

Outlier

This is quite different from rest of the data set. One should search for outliers in the data set.

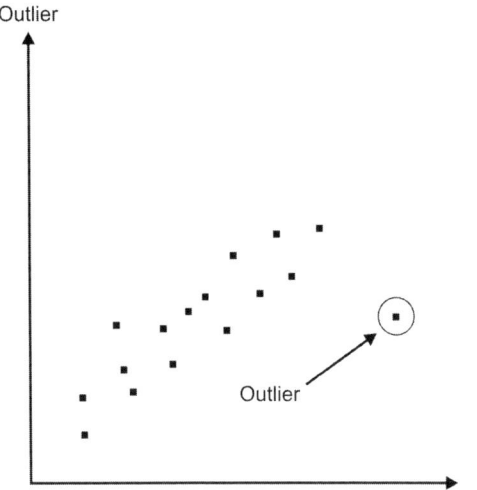

If not done, outliers can distort values and change statistical modeling as well.

Following are general rules of finding outliers:

a. If an observation has a value that is more than 2.5 times of the standard deviation from the mean.

b. Observation with a value, more than 1.5 times of inter-quartile range. This can be done using boxplot.

c. Do not discard outliers without a reason unless you find the cause of outliers. This may help us to understand cause of data variability.

P-value

This is called probability value or *p-value*. In hypothesis testing, this is the probability of getting a value at a set point is null hypothesis is true. If *p-value* is small, smaller then the set alpha value, null hypothesis is unlikely to be true and we have to select the alternative hypothesis.

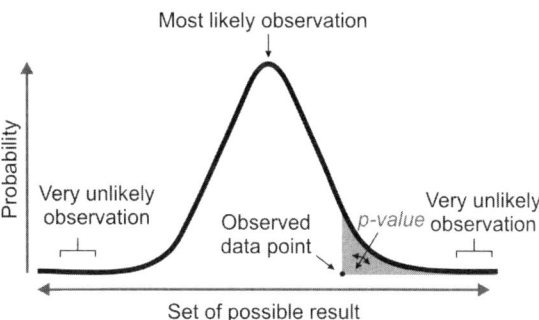

A *p-value* (shaded gray area) is the probability of an observed (or more extreme) result arising by chance

Parameter

This is the numerical value of a population. For example, blood pressure in men and women is more likely high compared to those below 50 years.

Population values are modeled from normal distribution and depend upon many parameters. For example, the parameters of the normal distribution from the population are the mean (μ) and the standard deviation (σ). For the binomial distribution, the parameters are the number of trials (n), and the probability of success (θ).

Pattern

Pattern is important in statistics and is expressed as:

Data = Pattern + residual

A good analysis will take into account all kind of patterns and pattern will take into consideration that data has variability and values could be different from each other. It is important to know that variability is the part of pattern or signal in the data. If some part of the data is not properly understood, it may form a part of "noise" and we may need to calculate signal/noise ratio. This in gross term is our "error".

In medical studies, outliers could be found and could form a part of "noise". A stated earlier, an outlier could be quite different from rest of the data set. One should search for outliers in the data set. If not done, outliers can distort values and change statistical modeling as well. Whole conclusions could be different in this case.

Percentage

How much out of 100 is called percent. For a variable, that has a (n) of observations and frequency of occurrence (r); percentage is calculated by the formula:

$$100 \times r/n$$

What percentage of patients coming to headache clinic have hypertension, if 20 out of 50 have increased blood pressure?

$$100 \times 20/50 = 40\%$$

Percentile

Percentile is the number indicating that at least percent of the values in the list are not larger than this. For example, if someone got a score of 99% percentile means, only 1% are above that score. Likewise, if someone has a score of 75% then there are 25% people have a score above that.

Population

This is the entire number of individuals of units that are under study. For example, when we have a census in India; then total number of people are studied.

Statistics is concerned with estimating population parameters from the sample statistics. Greek letters, e.g. μ, σ, θ are usually used for population parameters. This is to distinguish them from sample statistics, e.g. mean (X), standard deviation (s).

Precision

This is also called reliability and is related to standard error. Precision is a measure of how close an estimator is expected to be, to the true value of a parameter. This is usually expressed in terms of the standard error. Less precision is reflected by a larger standard error. If we want better precision, increase in sample size could be an option.

For example, if the sample mean, x, is used to estimate the population mean, μ, then the standard error (SE) is given by:

$$SE = \sigma/\sqrt{n}$$

σ is the standard deviation of the data

n is the sample size.

Decrease in standard error will improve precision and n has to be increased to decrease standard error.

Proportion

If frequency of observations is (r), and total number of observations are (n) then proportion (p) can be calculated as:

For example, what proportion of resident doctors plays tennis or cricket or go to gym in evening out of a total of 100 when the number of playing residents is 40?

As per formula ($p = r/n$)

$$40/100 = 0.4$$

If we multiply the same by 100%, results can be obtained in percentage.

Quantiles

These are a set of cut-off points that can be used to divide numerical variables into groups containing equal numbers of observations. Examples include quartiles, deciles, percentiles, etc.

Quartiles

The quartile is a number such that 1/4th of the values in the sorted list are not larger than it and at least 3/4th are not smaller than it.

Quintile

This is similar to quartile but divides the data into five sets. Therefore, the lowest quintile is the 20%.

Random Sample

This is an equal probability sample.

Range

Difference between highest and lowest value is called range. This is a very crude method of describing data distribution.

For example, average weight of children (3–5 years) coming to pediatric outpatient department in a given week is: 15 kg in one hospital and 20 kg in another.

Range could be given as 15–20 kg. (5 kg)

Risk

This is a very common expression in clinical medicine and epidemiological studies. Risk of event is basically a probability of that event occurring. For example, risk of occurring myocardial infarction in hypertensive men above the age of 50 years will be higher compared to young men between 35–45 years.

If absolute number of events could be 10 out of 100 men then the risk could be 0.1 or 10%.

Sample (Random Sample)

This is a group of units selected from a larger population. We always aim to draw valid conclusions by studying the sample. A sample is convenient as taking the whole population will be cumbersome and almost impossible. Many a times, if not, it is not desirable to study the whole group. Using laws of statistics, conclusions drawn from a small samples are applicable to population as a whole. This is called central limit theorem.

A sample has to be a random sample, that means, it defies chance and everyone has an equal probability of getting selected.

Sampling Distribution

When a random sample is drawn from the population; sampling distribution describes the probability associated with an estimator. The random sample just one the many sample. It is possible that each would give a different value for the estimator. The distribution of these different values is called the sampling distribution of estimator.

Deriving a sampling distribution is the first step in calculating a confidence interval or in performing hypothesis testing. Standard deviation of sampling distribution will tell us about the variability of estimator and is called standard error. Larger is sample size, smaller is standard error. That means, if the sample size is large the probability that it follows a normal distributor is high. This has been defined as per central limit theorem.

Mostly, 95% confidence intervals are judged by taking the value of mean ± 2 standard error.

Scatter Plot

Scatter plot consists of a display diagram and consists of a pair of values. The data is plotted as a series of point and if the data are ordered then it may be logical to join the successive points using a line. This then becomes a line graph.

If there are many categorical variables then their values can be indicated by using different symbols or colors.

Significance Level (Alpha Level) of a Hypothesis Test

This is a fixed probability of being wrong in statistical hypothesis testing and concluding that we wrongly rejected the null hypothesis (H_0).

If null hypothesis is true, then significance level is the probability alpha error and is set by the investigator right in beginning. Usually, the significance level is set at 0.05 (or equivalently, 5%).

Skewness of Data

Usually we deal with a data that is normally distributed. However, if the distribution of a variable is not symmetrical about the median or the mean it is said to be skewed data. The distribution has **positive skewness** if the tail of high values is longer than the tail of low values, and **negative skewness** if the reverse is true.

Spread, Measures

Data exhibits variability and naturally will have different type of values. If the data follows normal distribution; then one can have most of the data located around the centre and then towards the extreme end a thin amount of data is going to be located.

Spread of data will describe maximum and minimum data, inter-quartile range. Data spread can also be known by standard deviation.

Standard Deviation

This is a commonly used summary measure of spread of a data set. This is given along with mean. It is usually expressed as mean ± standard deviation. Most of the data (95%) will be within 2 standard deviations. Standard deviation is heavily influenced by the presence of outliers.

If the data value is like this: 12, 15, 11, 18, 13, 14, 18 and has a mean of 14.4.

The variance (σ^2) is 7.62, so the standard deviation, $\sigma = \sqrt{7.62} = 2.8$

The mean, x was 14.4, so $(x - \sigma) = (14.4 - 2.8) = 11.6$
and $(x + \sigma) = 17.2$

Standard Error (SE)

Just like standard deviation is a measure of spread of data set, standard error designated as SE is a measure of precision. This means, how close are your results to the real one in population and margin of error. It is a key concept in statistical inferences.

For example, if a survey is done in various Delhi hospitals about the smoking habits of health care workers; and a hypothetical value comes out to be 30% with standard error of 3%; then real value could be 33% or 27%. This helps us in calculating the confidence interval.

For example, 95% confidence interval will contain values within ± 2 SE. So confidence interval could be 30 – 6 = 24 and 30 + 6 = 36. That means, confidence interval for this finding that we have (i.e. 30%) will be 24 – 36. So that means true population proportion is likely to be anywhere between 24 and 36%.

Symmetrical

If the data values are distributed same way onto right side and left side of the mean; distribution is called symmetrical.

Such tests are easily interpreted and allow presence of outliers to be detected similarly. Some statistical tests are used only when tests are symmetrical and therefore transformation of asymmetrical data is sometimes done. Log values may help transform the data. Boxplot may be a good test to know about data symmetry or skewness, of a set of data.

Table

We use tables very frequently to describe and present data. Indeed tabulated data is much easier to handle compared to a haphazard data.

A data may be split into categories and a table provides a simple summary. A table may give frequency, or percentage and can help to summarize the data.

Test Statistic

Test statistic is a quantity calculated from the sample data and is used in hypothesis testing. Based upon the value of test statistics, null hypothesis could be rejected or not.

Which test statistic to be used depends upon the assumptions of models and hypothesis being tested. Mostly we compare means and

Table 1: Dinner dietary habits of some diabetic hypertensives	
Vegetarians	Non-vegetarians
Ice creams	Eggs (Fried)
6 chappatis	Chicken
Ghee	Butter Dal
Fried and salted vegetables	Peanuts

see if that difference is statistically significant, e.g. difference between observed and expected ($xE - x0$).

Time Series

This is a series of measurements overtime usually at regular intervals. That means this is a sequence of data points. Observations in this type of studies may be valuable in pattern recognition.

Transforming Variables

If the dataset we have shows evidence of skewness then transformation may lead to a more symmetrical distribution that could be amenable to many statistical tests.

Tukey

People working in statistics often use Honestly significant difference described by Tukey **(1915–2000)**, a Chemistry graduate and a statistician from Princeton University. "Bits" for computer word was coined by him and later on in 1970 he introduced boxplot.

Variable

This is an observed or measured characteristic like blood pressure, heart rate, hours of sunlight exposure per day, etc. they may be numerical or non-numerical or categorical.

Average or mean is used to quantify the numerical variables while a table of frequencies or percentages may be used to summarize a categorical variable.

Variability in Data

If there are many different values in a given data set, then we can conclude that the data shows lot of variation. Too much of variability can actually make it difficult to differentiate "signal from noise". It can be measured by variance (*see* below).

Variance

Variance is a measure of variability and is denoted by σ^2 and the square root of variance is called standard deviation. This is more often used as it can be applied to both sides of data and as same units as mean. Therefore it is easy to interpret. It could be useful when contribution from different sources are assessed and Analysis of Variance (ANOVA) is very popular method of comparing differences between 3 or more means.

It is calculated by the formula

$$\sigma^2 = \Sigma(x - x)2/(n - 1)$$

Zero Values in a Data Set

Presence of zero in a data set may be there and could be modeled separately if needed.

Appendix 2
Commonly Used Terms in Clinical Trials

Active Comparator

This is an active drug that could be used to compare the results with a test drug.

This is one of the several arms that a clinical trial may have, e.g. a placebo arm.

Active but not Recruiting

This is a type of clinical study that is active or is ongoing but is not currently recruiting participants in clinical trials.

Adverse Drug Events or Adverse Events

This could be a favorable change in health condition of the participant during clinical trial. This could also occur after sometime of the study period as some of the adverse events may have delayed onset. It should be noted that the events may not always be caused by the drugs per se.

AGREEMENTS

Many agreements has to be an agreements between the principal investigator (PI) and the sponsor of the trial that prohibits, the PI to discuss the results of the study or to publish the study results in a scientific or academic journal after the trial is completed.

Allocation in Clinical Trials

This is a clinical trial design in which participants are assigned a particular arm in clinical trial, e.g. placebo arm or treatment arm. Allocation could be randomized or non-randomized.

Arm in a Trial

An arm is a group of subgroup that is participating in a clinical trial and may receive a drug or the placebo as per the standard trial protocol. Arm has to be decided before the trial begins. Further description of the arm could be given and arm in a clinical trial may include: experimental or treatment arm, placebo comparator arm, sham surgery arm and no intervention arm.

BASELINE CHARACTERISTICS

This is the data set recorded in the beginning of a clinical study or trial and is done for all participants. Same set is to be repeated for comparison or reference group also.

Data collected could include age, sex, and study related measures, such as blood pressure, heart rate. A history of prior disease should be taken as per inclusion and exclusion criteria.

Blinding

When we conduct clinical trial, doctor and patient should have no information about what one is taking. This is called double blinding. Nowadays, "triple blinding" is also encouraged to ensure that the statistician that is involved in analysis of data has no idea about the data set and is able to analyze the same without prejudice or personal bias.

Clinical Study

This is a research study that uses human beings to evaluate the effect of drug/s in human beings. These could be interventional (e.g. a drug being evaluated) or non-interventional or observational study. Former type of studies are also called clinical trials.

Clinical Trials

In this type of study, usually a drug is compared against the placebo or psychological medicine to see if the drug has the active component and is having better efficacy. Placebo is acting as a control here. In uncontrolled trials, the possibility of bias is more as there is no comparison group against which the effect of the drug in question can be compared.

Clinical Trial Registry

This is clinical trial code that is given by clinical register in India. Any clinical trial before it enrolls the first patient should have the clinical trial registered here. This is to ensure transparency in India. Trial registration has started after the year 2009 and is now mandatory. Biomedical journals in India do not accept a paper for publication in a journal until the trial has a registration number. This information is present in public domain.

Clinical Research Organizations (CROs)

This is particularly common in India and there are over 100 CROs in India. So clinical research in India is a booming industry and is growing at an annual rate of 30%.

Closed Studies

These are kind of studies that are no longer recruiting patients. Its like saying "House-full", no more vacancies, i.e. enough number of participants are already there. A trial terminated for whatever reason may also be termed a "closed study".

At some websites, it appears as RED text showing that the trial is no more interested in taking patients.

Table 1: Some of the commonly used terms for "closed trials"

Active, but not recruiting
Completed or terminated
Suspended or withdrawn
Enrolling by invitation only
Temporarily not available
No longer available for expanded access
Trial completed and the drug approved for marketing

Collaborator

This is an organization that provides support for clinical trials. In india, this is mostly done by Clinical Research Organizations (CROs).

This therefore is an organization that is not the sponsor.

Completed Study

This is a type of study that has stopped recruiting as the drug either has been approved and study completed or the study completed long ago but the drug is under consideration for approval.

Condition (Clinical)

This is a disease or disorder or a syndrome or illness or any other health related issue important in clinical trials.

Controlled Trial

This is a type of clinical trial in which the observations about the test drug are compared to a standard (called control). Standard may be from the same trial or from some different trial conducted earlier. This may then be referred as "historical" control.

Crossover Design

This is a clinical trial in which the participants receive two or more interventions in a particular order. The group that was earlier receiving the placebo, now receives the drug and vice versa. So during the study period, "there is a crossing over". Important feature of this type of trial is that all participants are receiving the drugs at a given point of time.

Data Monitoring Committee

This is a group of independent clinical trial professionals or who monitor drug safety and scientific standards of a trial. The group can:
   a. Recommend stopping the trial if it is not effective.
   b. Not scientific enough.

Members are chosen based upon their expertise and scientific skills. In some countries, they are labeled as data safety monitoring boards.

Double Blinding

Double blinding is a type of masking in which doctors and patients are not aware about what interventions have been assigned to what group, i.e. drug and placebo. Even the statistician involved in analysis should not have any idea about the hypothesis and other study details like aims and objective to ensure complete blinding (triple blinding).

Eligibility Criteria

These are study standards set right in beginning that participants who are enrolled in study must meet to ensure their participation. These include inclusion and exclusion criteria. They should not be too narrow else external validity gets affected.

Enrollment

Normally, participants may be selected from groups, or population but they could also be enrolled by invitation. This form of participation is decided in advance. Such studies are not opened to anyone who meets eligibility criteria but only to people particular to that population.

Enrollment in Clinical Study

This is a procedure in which the participants are registered for the study whose aim, objectives, and duration have been specified.

Exclusion Criteria

It means, subject/s is/are not fit for study. This has to be very clear as failure to exclude improper patient may limit sample size and we may lose vital information about the same.

Expanded Access

This is a process put in place by drug regulatory authorities to allow manufacturers to provide Investigational New Drugs (INDs) to the patients with serious conditions who otherwise cannot participate in clinical trials.

Experimental Arm

This is also called test arm, this arm contains the active drug under study.

Factorial Design

This is a type of study in which participants receive one of the several combinations of interventions. This enables clinical researchers to evaluate more than 1 treatments at one time. At a simple level, 2×2 study design is chosen in which 2 different treatments at two different levels are involved. Same group of patients are re-used here. For example, if there is a clinical trial that involves aspirin and placebo for reducing risk of ischemic heart disease; then same patients can be given ticlopidine and placebo in a crossover fashion.

Food and Drug Administration (FDA)

Food and Drug Administration (FDA) is an agency regulating public health by ensuring the safety and efficacy of drugs, vaccines and other biological products. FDA maintains a portal in India so that products getting exported from India meet global standards.

Funding Agency

This is an agency describing funding sources for the clinical study. In India these may include Department of Biotechnology, Indian Council of Medical Research and Central Scientific and Industrial Research (CSIR), etc.

Private funding may also come via pharmaceutical companies also as a research grant.

Gender Eligibility

Both males and females could be recruited in the study for purpose of evaluating a drug.

HEALTH AUTHORITY

This could be a national or international authority that has control over the clinical trial being conducted. Directorate General Health Services and Drug (DGHS) Controller General of India (DGI) are such bodies in India.

Human Study Subjects Review Board (Institute Review Board in India)

Ethical approval for any clinical research study is a must if it involves, "More than minimal harm" to the participants. Often, ethical committee believes that researchers are not in position to determine this. Therefore, taking ethical approval will always be handy. So, this is commonly called Institution Ethical Committee (IEC) or alternatively Institutional Review Board (IRB).

A group of people will review, approve or monitor the clinical study protocol and then formally approve the study. Their role is to protect the rights and welfare of human beings in research study.

This will involve a heterogeneous group like an advocate, scientist, medical doctor, administrator and even a layman.

Inclusion

These are a group of conditions that are set in beginning based upon which entry of the study subject in clinical trial is ensured. Also called entry criteria.

Informed Consent

This is a process of taking acceptance from the study participants regarding enrollment in a clinical study.

There are preconditions and methodology that needs to be explained to patients:

Rules for Taking Informed Consent

a. Provide all information about the study so that the participant can make an informed choice about whether to remain in the study or go out.

b. Risks and benefits of participation in study should be explained and it should be emphasized that the participation is totally voluntary.

c. Saying yes in a clinical study is NOT a contract and participation is free to leave the study anytime. Importantly, this will have no bearing with the drug treatment.

d. Goal of informed consent is to protect study participants and allay anxieties about the research.

e. Document must be simple, easy to read and written in a clear language.

f. A person/subject signing the consent form becomes enrolled in the study.

g. No force, coercion or greed should be offered to the participant.

Intervention

This is usually a drug or a placebo or any device or procedure that is under clinical study. These could be assigned as single group design, parallel group design (most common), crossover design and factorial design.

INTERVENTIONAL STUDY (CLINICAL TRIAL)

Interventional study is a type of clinical study in which participants are assigned to receive one or more intervention on biomedical or health related outcomes. Assigning what to whom depends and varies as per study protocol and participants may receive diagnostic, therapeutic or some other type of intervention. Cf observational study.

Investigational New Drug (IND)

This is a drug or a biological product that is used in clinical trial but has not been formally approved by a drug regulatory authority.

Investigator in a Clinical Trial

This is a scientifically trained research that is involved in clinical study. Principal investigator the lead investigator and is also called study director. Co-Principal Investigator (Co-PI) works in close collaboration with principal investigator.

Masking

This is a clinical trial strategy in which participants and investigators are not aware about who is receiving what. This is also called blinding.

Double blinding is the most common type and is a type of masking in which doctors and patients are not aware about what interventions have been assigned to what group, i.e. drug and placebo. Even the statistician involved in analysis should not have any idea about the hypothesis and other study details like aims and objective to ensure complete blinding (triple blinding). Open label is another form of study in which doctors and patients know what is being given to whom.

Non-intervention Arm

This is an arm in which participants do not receive any intervention during a clinical study. This may be one of the several arms.

Observational Study

This is a type of clinical study in which there is no intervention. Participants are just assessed for health related outcomes and analyzed. They may receive therapeutic, diagnostic or any other type of interventions but they are not assigned by a clinical trial investigator. These could be Cohort, case control studies. Some of the variations may include case only (case reports), case series, case-crossover, ecological or community based studies.

Open Label Study

This is a type of study frequently done in India. A distinguishing feature is that masking is not used and both trial investigator and patients know who is taking what.

Open Label Extension

When a trial is concluded, all information is subjected to the regulatory authority for approval of drug. However, in some cases, the drug is given to participants and codes are broken (i.e. there is no blinding). Properly designed open label extension studies can give valuable information about the drug in terms of its efficacy. Compromise on research ethics is a potential drawback. These follow the double blind study of a new drug.

OPEN STUDIES

These are studies that are currently recruiting. Various types of status could be:

• Recruiting
• Not yet recruiting
• Expanded access

Parallel Design

This is a trial in which two or more groups of participants receive different interventions. In a two arm parallel design, one group receives placebo and other receives the test drug. Later on, it can be swapped and it becomes a parallel and crossover design.

Phases of Clinical Trials

Phase 0: This is a type of exploratory studies, also called micro-dose studies or screening studies.

Phase 1: These are studies conducted in human volunteers aimed at finding the maximally tolerated dose, safety and any serious adverse events. Main goal is to know pharmacokinetic details.

Phase 2: These are done to generate the priliminary data on drug efficacy. This is done in patients. It can be done with placebo or active comparator. Short-term adverse effects may also be found.

Phase 3: These are studies that generate lot of other details about efficacy and may refute null hypothesis. These are generally blinded and controlled. Additional safety data gets generated as these are done in larger number of patients.

Phase 4: Also called post-marketing surveillance or adverse drug reaction monitoring. This can generate data on safety, and efficacy of the drug.

PLACEBO

This is a "psychological medicine" that is similar to original drug in taste, packing, smell and presentation, etc. This is to mask any differences that two drugs may have.

PRIMARY OUTCOME MEASURE

This is the major planned outcome of the study and is very important. This may be CT scan or MRI brain or any blood parameter. It may also be a clinical endpoint measured by a scale. It may be one or more.

PRIMARY AIM

This is the main reason doing a clinical study or trial. It may be a diagnostic, or therapeutic.

PRINCIPAL INVESTIGATOR (PI)

This is the main person responsible for scientific and technical direction of study. Co-principal investigator assists the PI in doing the same.

PROTOCOL

This is a written detail of the study and may include aims, objectives, study design, material, methods, timeline, etc. It should have clear description of statistical methods.

PUBLICATIONS

Any scientific article of abstract about a clinical study or a trial.

Radom Allocation

A strategy by which the participants are allocated to different arms.

RECRUITMENT STATUS

This means whether a study is available for recruitment or is closed.

REGISTRATION

This is the process of submitting information about a clinical study or a trial to a public registry. Indian Clinical Trial registry is there in India.

REGISTRY

This is a structured online system for maintaining database of clinical trial and could provide information both to public and trial investigators. It could contain information about both ongoing and completed trials.

REPORTING GROUP

This is a comparison group of participants that is used for summarizing data in a clinical trials.

Result Database

This is a structured online system that may provide a public portal for clinical trials. Indian Clinical Trial registry is one such attempt by Indian Council of Medical Research.

Secondary Outcome Measure

This is a planned outcome measure in clinical trial protocol that is not as important as the primary outcome measure but still has been keeping trial and requirements in mind. Most of the studies may have more than one primary objective.

It is important to know that the sample size is calculated keeping only the primary objective in mind. Secondary objective does not count towards sample size calculations.

Serious Adverse Events

This is an adverse event that may result into hospitalization, a life-threatening event or results in death or disability. They could even be considered to be the serious adverse events if they put the participants in a life-threatening situation.

Sham Arm (Comparator)

This is a group of participants that receive an intervention that is very similar to that of the original one, but is not the real one. It should be as close to real as is possible.

SINGLE BLIND MASKING

A type of masking in which one party involved with the clinical trial, either the investigator or participant, does not know which participants have been assigned which interventions.

SINGLE GROUP DESIGN

Describes a clinical trial in which all participants receive the same intervention. One type of Intervention Model Design.

SPONSOR (LEAD OR MAIN)

This is an organization or the person who is overseeing the data or is analyzing the same.

Sponsor-investigator

Person who is financing the clinical trial and/or is also the lead investigator.

STATUS

Generally refer to recruitment status.

Study Start and Completion Date

The date by which the participants have made their first visit and they have been recruited. The date by which the study participants have made their final visit to the site of study.

Study Design

This refers to various tools that investigators use during the course of study. These may be the primary purpose, intervention design, masking and allocation, etc.

Study Records

This is an official entry of the data which is kept during and after the study is over. Study data has to be stored for a reasonable period. Safe locker facilities are available nowadays for better data storage.

Study Type

This refers to the type of study: Observational, interventional or expanded excess, etc.

SUSPENDED

This is a study that has been stopped but may start again.

Terminated

This is a study that has been stopped and will not start again.

Time Frame

This is a sequence of events that are to be specified in clinical trials and one has to be clear about starting date, completion dates and major milestones, etc.

Title of Clinical Trial

Nowadays, there is a trend of using acronyms for clinical trial. For example, Clinical Trial of Antipsychotic Effectiveness and Intervention (CATIE) trial was done to compare safety and efficacy of older verses new antipsychotics.

UNKNOWN RECRUITMENT STATUS

It is a type of clinical study in which the status of recruitment has not been specified. These could be open or closed studies depending upon their last recruitment status.

Withdrawn

A clinical study that has been stopped before enrolling its first participant.

Index